Hope and Destiny, Jr.

THE ADOLESCENT'S GUIDE TO SICKLE CELL DISEASE

REVISED THIRD EDITION

Lewis L. Hsu, MD
Carmen C. M. Rodrigues, RN
Silvia R. Brandalise, MD

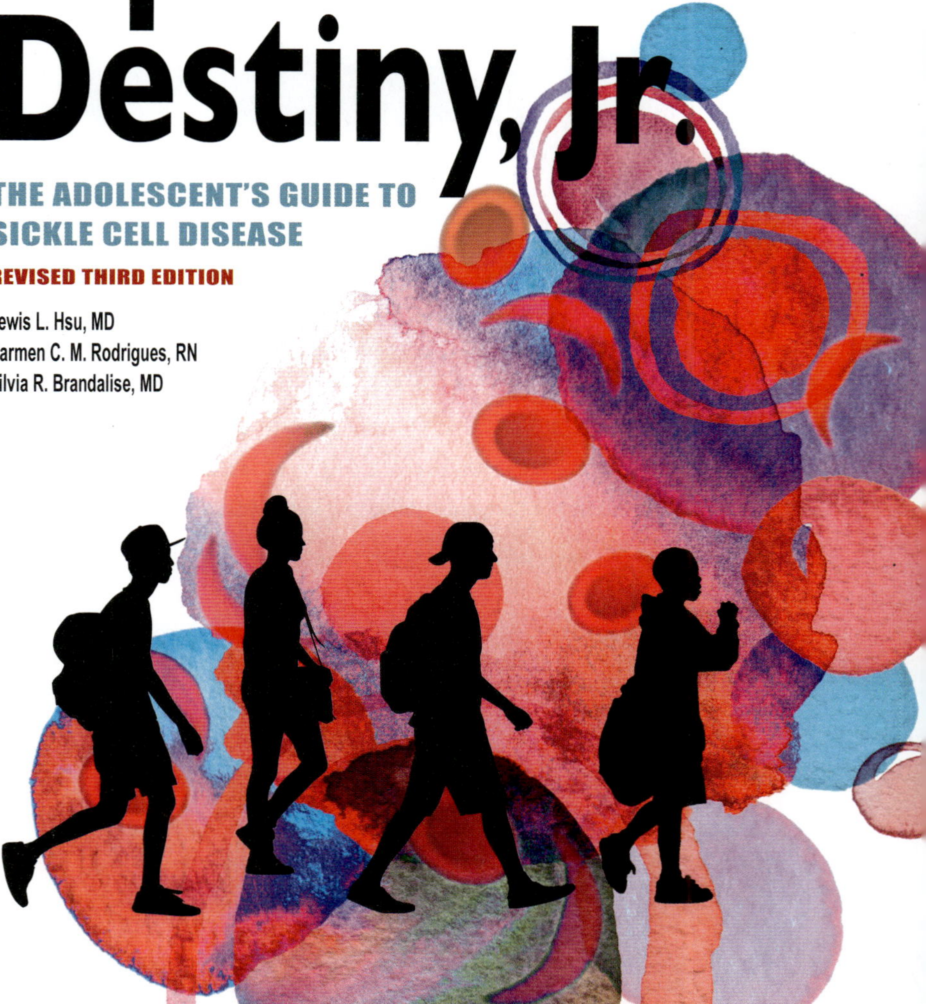

HILTON PUBLISHING
Hilton Publishing · Chicago, Illinois

Hilton Publishing Company
Chicago, IL

Direct all correspondence to:
Hilton Publishing Company
5261 Fountain Drive, Suite A
Crown Point, IN 46307
219–922–4868
www.hpcinternationalinc.com

ISBN 978-0-9773160-5-2

Notice: The information in this book is true and complete to the best of the authors' and publishers' knowledge. This book is intended only as an information reference and should not replace, countermand, or conflict with the advice given to readers by their physicians. The authors and publisher disclaim all liability in connection with the specific personal use of any and all information provided in this book.

Angela Vennemann, Senior Editor and Design
Megan Lippert, Executive Vice President, Hilton Publishing Division

Original illustrations by Tifani Carter

The Library of Congress has cataloged the 2016 printing as follows:

Library of Congress Cataloging-in-Publication Data

Hsu, Lewis.
The adolescent's guide to sickle cell diseases / Lewis Hsu, M.D.
pages cm
Audience: Grade 7 to 8.
ISBN 978-0-9764443-1-2
1. Sickle cell anemia—Juvenile literature. 2. Genetic disorders—Juvenile literature. I. Title.
RC641.7.S5H78 2013
616.1'527—dc23
2013007369

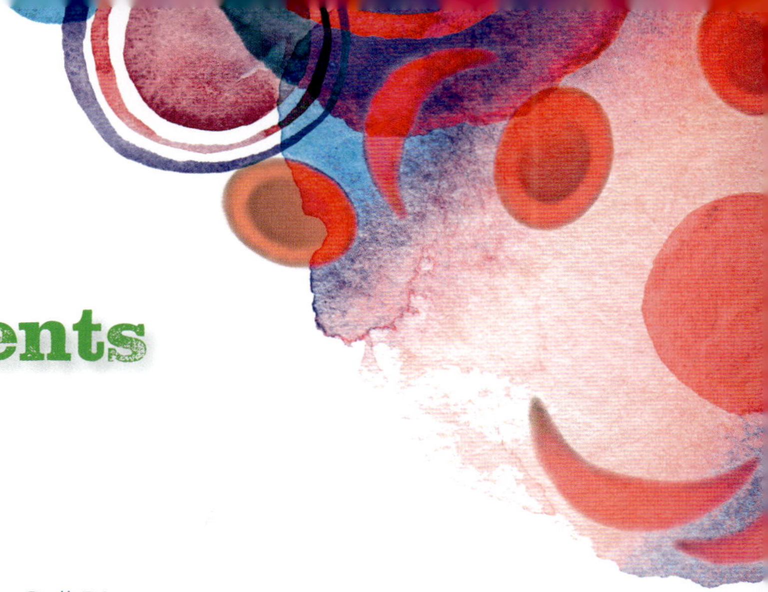

TABLE OF Contents

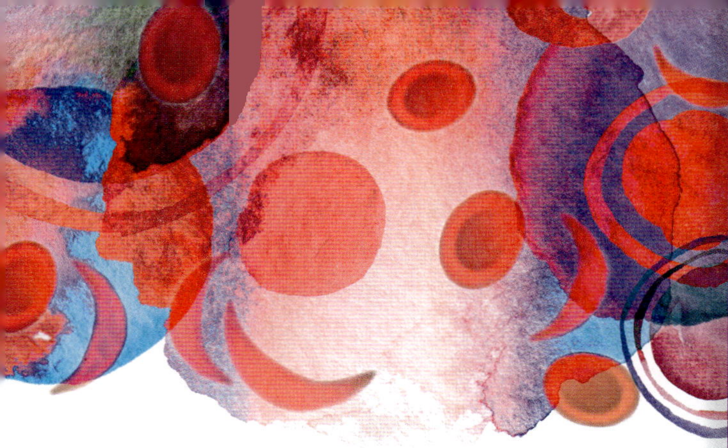

Do things you always thought you couldn't do.

—Samone, teen with SCD

SECTION 1

HISTORY OF Sickle Cell Disease

THE STORY OF WALTER CLEMENT NOEL

Sickle cell disease was first described in Chicago, Illinois, just over 100 years ago.

Walter Clement Noel finished his schooling in Grenada, a small island nation in the southeastern Caribbean Sea, but he wanted to continue his education so he could become a dentist. There were only two dentists practicing in all of Grenada. He found out that Chicago was one of the few places that would train Black men in dentistry.

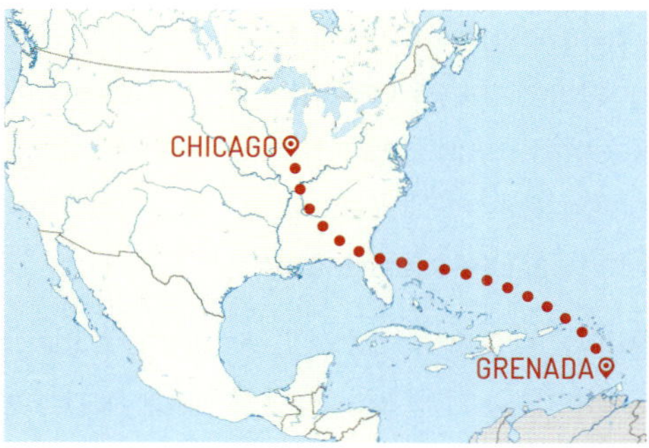

His mother was worried about letting him go to Chicago. Why? Because it was more than 2,500 miles away, and he would be a foreigner in a big city. Chicago was known for being a busy industrial city, and it had no palm trees! She heard that Chicago had beaches but that the sun was not as warm as in Grenada, and sometimes it was windy and snowy. Sometimes it was so cold that the lakes and rivers froze. Nothing ever froze in Grenada. But Walter was determined. He applied to the Chicago College of Dental Surgery and was accepted. His mother wrote a letter to the head of the dental school, asking him to look out for Walter.

Walter took a ship from Grenada to America. The trip took a week and he got seasick (Today it is an airplane ride of about five hours, and nobody gets seasick—but maybe airsick). He landed at Ellis Island, near the Statue of Liberty in New York Harbor on September 14, 1904. At Ellis Island, all the travelers had to show that they were healthy enough to enter the United States. Walter had some sores on his legs and wondered if the doctor would let him continue on to Chicago so that he could fulfill his dream of becoming a dentist.

Documents from Ellis Island in New York show that Walter traveled to the U.S. on a ship called the Cearense. The ship's manifest records that Walter was in good health, possessed $70.00 in cash, and was "Going to study Dentistry in the College" in Chicago.

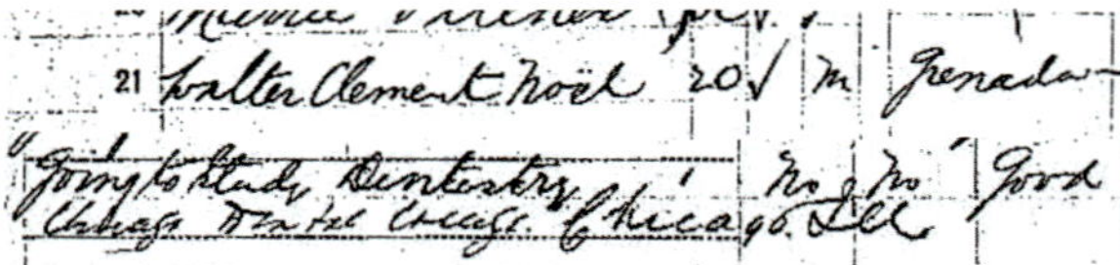
21 Walter Clement Noel 20 m Grenada
Going to study Dentistry Chicago Dental College Chicago Ill No No Good

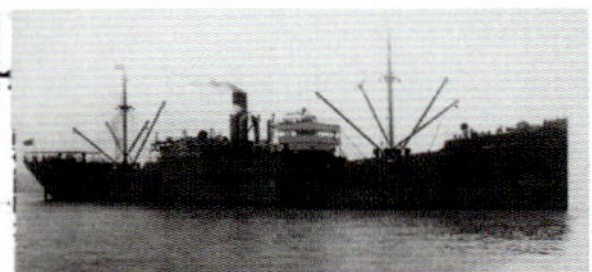

Everybody sat in a long line waiting to be examined by the Ellis Island doctor. The doctor examined Walter quickly and found the sores on his legs but did not think they were a problem. He recommended some iodine treatment to keep the skin clean and let Walter into the United States. Soon Walter was on his way to Chicago. He started dental school right near where the Illinois Medical District is today.

While in dental school, Walter got sick several times with strange pains. Sometimes his legs or his back hurt, and doctors thought it was arthritis. Sometimes his chest hurt, and doctors thought it was an infection in his lungs. Cold weather brought on more of these problems, and the pains got especially bad in the severe winters of Chicago. The winter of 1905 saw record-setting cold and snow, and Walter was in the hospital a lot. His doctors could not figure out what was causing his problems, but they gave him morphine to help ease the pain.

One young doctor, Ernest E. Irons, had the bright idea to do a new test on Walter's blood. He looked at a thin layer of Walter's blood under the microscope. Dr. Irons was very surprised to find "cells of an unusual elongated shape" and showed them to his professor, James B. Herrick. They could not figure out why Walter's cells looked this way, but they realized it was something new and not just arthritis or pneumonia. Each time Walter was hospitalized, Dr. Irons took notes on what happened and discussed it with Dr. Herrick. Finally, Dr. Herrick wrote a medical paper describing this new disease. Other doctors began to recognize it in their patients when they looked under the microscope at their blood. They named it sickle cell disease because the long shape and sharp pointed tips of the red blood cells reminded them of a farming tool called a sickle.

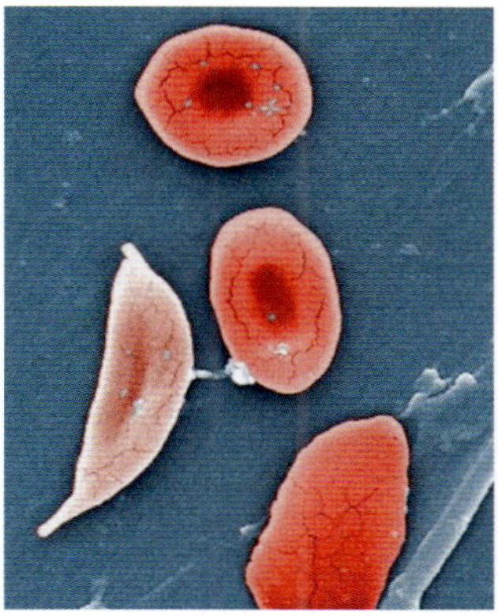

These are all red blood cells, but the one on the left is a sickled red blood cell.

What happened to Walter Clement Noel? There was a name for his disease but not much treatment. He learned that staying warm and drinking a lot of liquids kept his body stronger and helped him avoid some of the painful episodes. He studied hard, and the head of the dental school helped him catch up on the work he missed each time he was hospitalized. He graduated from dental school in 1907.

The new Dr. Noel went back to Grenada on another ocean steamship voyage and was greeted by his proud mother. He was now a full-fledged dentist, only the third dentist in all of Grenada. The other two dentists were happy to have somebody join them in taking care of people's teeth and guided

Acute chest syndrome

Acute chest syndrome is a type of sickle cell crisis involving the lungs, and it can prevent your lungs from bringing enough oxygen into your bloodstream. Symptoms include fever, cough, difficulty breathing, and chest pain. Acute chest syndrome can be very dangerous, so if you have these symptoms, you should seek medical attention.

him along as he created his dental practice in Georgetown, the capital of Grenada. He did well and worked as a respected dentist for years.

At around age 33, as Walter traveled a full day to see a horse race, he got wet in the rain. He developed chest pain and lung problems which caused him to have difficulty breathing, and then rapidly got worse and soon died of what we commonly know today is called sickle cell acute chest syndrome. He is buried in his family cemetery in Grenada.

From the very first recognized case, people have been overcoming sickle cell disease with the support of family, such as Walter Noel's proud mother, and friends, such as the head of the Chicago College of Dental Surgery.

SICKLE CELL DISEASE IN AFRICA

WHY WAS SICKLE CELL DISEASE NOT DESCRIBED FIRST IN AFRICA?

The main reasons are because African people did not publish medical papers, and because there was no way to look at blood under a microscope to see the sickle shapes until the late 1800s. Most people born with sickle cell disease died as babies or young children and were typically not seen by physicians.

The first reports of sickle cell in African medical literature were in the 1870s. This may be because the symptoms were similar to those of other tropical diseases and because blood was not usually examined.

WHAT DID PEOPLE IN AFRICA CALL SICKLE CELL DISEASE?

African tribal populations did know of a disease that caused terrible pain. They named the disease in their own languages. Many tribal names describe a painful condition with names like "body chewing" or "body biting." Other names seem to be imitations of the cries and moans of the sufferers.

It is interesting to note that the tribal names have repeating syllables—possibly to symbolize the repeating painful episodes.

Here are other names for sickle cell disease from tribes around Ghana:

* ahututuo (from the Twi tribe)
* chwecheechwe (from the Ga tribe)
* nuidudui (from the Ewe tribe)
* nwiiwii (from the Fante tribe)

In one West African tribe, children who died soon after birth were called "ogbanjes," meaning children who come and go. The people believed that an evil spirit was trying to be born into a family with ogbanje children, but the babies bravely died to save the rest of the family from the demon.[1]

WHAT IS SICKLE CELL DISEASE?

Sickle cell disease is a common blood disorder someone is born with, where red blood cells form into a hard banana shape instead of being their normal, soft, round donut shape. As blood cells travel throughout the body, they all have important jobs to do. Red blood cells are in charge of carrying oxygen throughout the body, white blood cells help fight infections, and platelets help stop bleeding when you get a cut or scrape. For someone with sickle cell disease, the sickled red blood cells can easily get stuck trying to move through the body and can cause a sort of traffic jam, making it difficult for other healthy blood cells to keep moving through the body.

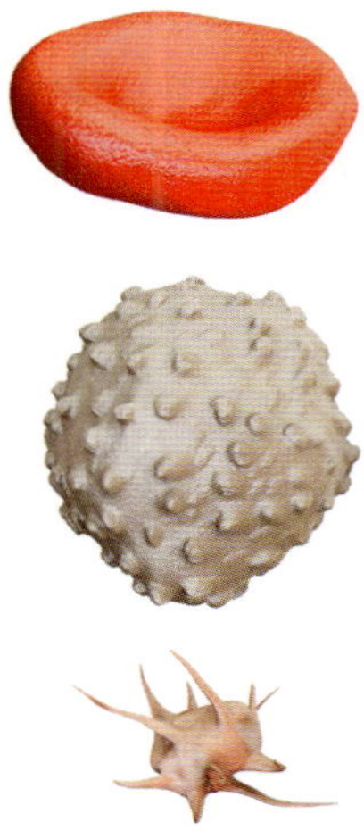

iStock / Getty Images

Top to bottom: red blood cell, white blood cell, and platelet

1 *http://innvista.com/health/ailments/anemias/sickle-cell-history/*

Just like a water pipe getting clogged in your house, this clogging of blood cells causes all kinds of very serious problems inside a person's body, such as pain where the blood cells get stuck, difficulty breathing from the body not getting enough oxygen, being unable to fight off infections as easily, and many other problems.

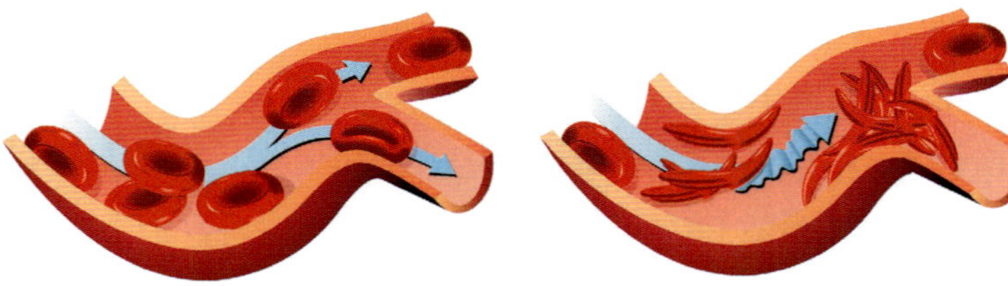

Healthy red cells move easily. Sickled red cells can get stuck.

SICKLE CELL DISEASE AND HEMOGLOBIN

Hemoglobin is the red protein that fills up red blood cells and allows it to carry oxygen from the lungs throughout the rest of the body. The abbreviation for hemoglobin is Hb or Hgb. Hemoglobin normally floats around inside the red blood cell as individual molecules. When a person has sickle cell disease, sickle hemoglobin can stack up (polymerizes) forming long solid sticks that change the shape of the red blood cell, causing it to sickle. Losing oxygen is the usual trigger for the red blood cell to change shape. Other reasons are dehydration or buildup of body acid.

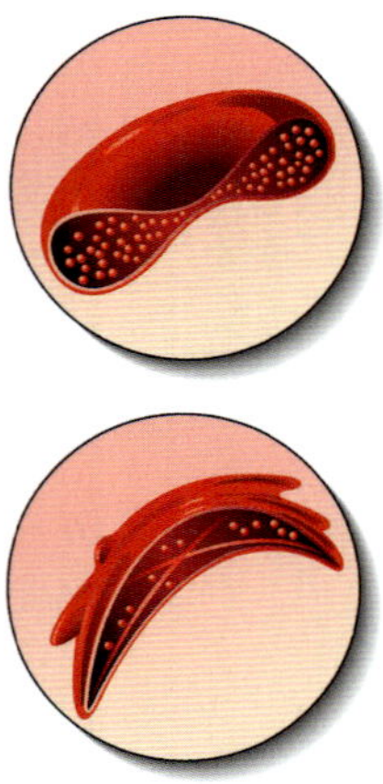

Top: typical hemoglobin
Bottom: polymerized hemoglobin that causes the sickle shape

Doctors commonly perform blood tests, taking a small sample of a person's blood to check how much hemoglobin, white blood cells and blood chemistry like glucose (sugar) they find in the blood. Some types of blood tests detect what type of hemoglobin is present, and this test could reveal a problem, like sickle cell disease.

Today in the United States a simple blood test is performed on most babies just after they are born, to check if their blood is healthy and if they have any medical conditions the parents should be aware of. Different states and hospitals do things a little differently, but most hospitals check every baby for these conditions in their newborn screening program, using a blood test and other evaluations:

* **sickle cell disease**
* **phenylketonuria (PKU)**—a genetic disorder that causes a type of acid to build up in the body, leading to seizures, developmental delays, behavioral problems, and psychiatric disorders
* **cystic fibrosis (CF)**—a genetic disorder that causes a buildup of thick, sticky mucus in the body. The most common symptoms are damage to the lungs and problems with the digestive system.
* **critical congenital heart disease**—serious heart defects that are present at birth
* **hearing loss**

HOW DO KIDS GET SCD?

SICKLE CELL DISEASE IS HEREDITARY

There are different types of sickle cell disease, and the type someone has depends on who else in their family has passed it along to them through genes. Genes are passed down from a parent to a child and make up the instructions that determine your body's traits, such as eye color, blood type, and disease risks. When a condition is passed from a parent to their child, we call it hereditary—meaning the child inherited the condition directly from one or both parents. When a condition results from a change or problem in the genes that make up our DNA, we call it a genetic disorder. Sickle cell disease is an example of a genetic disorder. If you have sickle cell disease, you have inherited it from your parents, and you may pass it along to any children you have when you grow up. If you receive only one sickle cell gene, then you have sickle cell trait, or SCT.

There are different types of hemoglobin, and the way the genes for these types are combined can cause different types of sickle cell disease. Typical

A Punnett square is a tool you can use to determine the possibility of inheriting a certain genetic condition. Everyone has two copies of a hemoglobin gene—one from each parent. Here's an example: if both of your parents have sickle trait (one gene for hemoglobin type A and one for type S) you have a one-in-four chance of having sickle cell disease (SS type).

Mom's hemoglobin genes

Dad's hemoglobin genes	A	S
A	**AA** (healthy hemoglobin)	**AS** (sickle trait)
S	**AS** (sickle trait)	**SS** (sickle cell disease)

hemoglobin is usually type A, while sickle hemoglobin is type S.

In the most common type of sickle cell disease in the United States and most countries, the gene for sickle hemoglobin is inherited from both parents and results in the production of only abnormal sickle hemoglobin. This is called sickle cell disease, SS type. It is also called sickle cell anemia.

The same sickling of red blood cells shows up in lesser-known forms of the disease as well. The SC type, often called "SC disease," and sickle beta thalassemia, or "S beta thal" or "sickle beta thal," are quite common. In sickle cell disease SC, one parent passes down the gene for sickle hemoglobin, while the other parent contributes the gene for type C hemoglobin, another abnormal hemoglobin type.

Similarly, a child with S beta thal also has one gene that makes sickle hemoglobin. But the other half of the equation, the beta thalassemia gene, produces either poorly functioning hemoglobin or none at all. In this situation, the majority—if not all—of the resulting hemoglobin is sickle hemoglobin.

There are other types of sickle cell disease that are rarer: SO-Arab, SD-Punjab or SD-Los Angeles, and others. While certain differences mark each of these syndromes, the resulting symptoms are quite similar.

It's important to note that sickle cell disease results not only from the inheritance of two sickle hemoglobin genes, but also from one sickle hemoglobin gene combined with another abnormal hemoglobin gene. If you decide to have children one day, this is something you will need to discuss with your partner and possibly with the help of a genetic counselor.

STORIES FROM KIDS LIKE YOU

I found out about sickle cell disease when I was four years old. Before we knew what the disease was, I had had several mild crises, such as pain and swelling. When I was six years old, I had my first violent crisis. It was then we discovered why I was suffering so much. After that, from September 2006 to April 2010, I was in the hospital every three months suffering many crises and taking continuous doses of morphine, Tramal, Tylex, aspirin, Lisador, dipyrone, Alivium, and so on. It was a cocktail to ease the intense pain that was crossing my whole body, not to mention unaccountable blood transfusions. Every crisis was accompanied with pneumonia. During this period, I also underwent surgery for a hernia and a gallbladder. I could not do any type of physical exertion. I could not run, jump, ride a bike, nor have any kind of fun. Everything resulted in returning to the hospital. In April 2010, I was taken to the Boldrini Center in São Paolo, Brazil. At the first consultation I was started on Hydrea, a wonderful medicine that saved my life. It completely changed my way of life. Since then, I have never felt any pain. I am another person. I was able to develop myself both physically and mentally. I still have be in treatment every three months, but I am living another life. I'm so happy. I do physical education at school, ride my bike, run and do everything, within my limits, of course. My eating habits have changed 100% and they are much healthier. Today I can truly be thankful for my treatment. I appreciate all the attention, care and affection that I have received and which has changed my life.

Herick, 12 years old

It's important that my child understands how to "read" the signs of her body in order to minimize a crisis.

—Myesha, parent

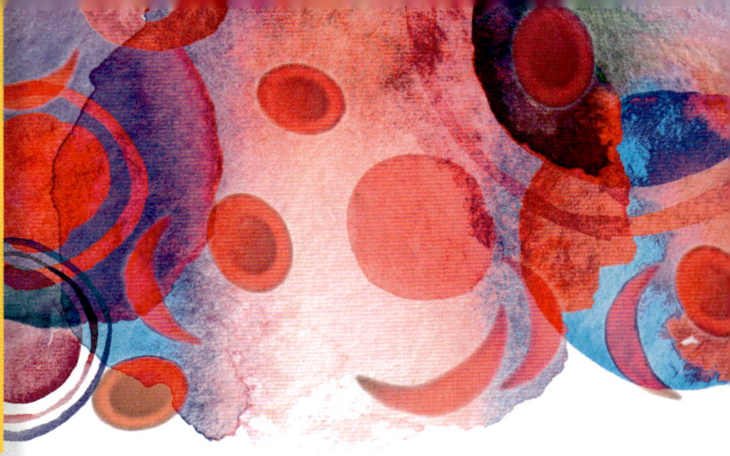

SECTION 2

TREATING AND PREVENTING Problems

TIPS FOR KEEPING YOUR BODY HEALTHY

People with sickle cell must drink plenty of fluids. Water is the best choice; milk or juice is next best. Do not take in too much coffee, tea or caffeinated drinks—these drinks don't help your body retain as much water, which can cause you to become dehydrated more easily. Plus, too many sugary carbonated soft drinks are bad for your teeth.

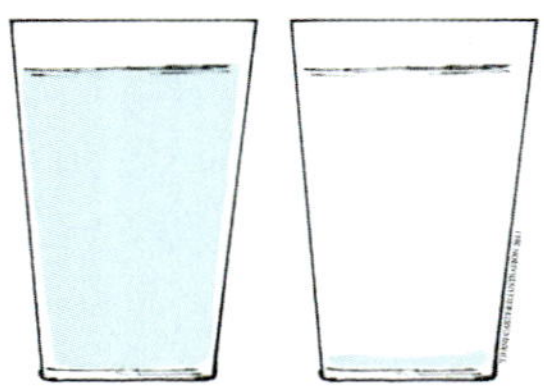

Water is the best choice for staying hydrated.

Folic acid, which is in the B-vitamin group, can help people with sickle cell disease make red blood cells and might also help keep their blood vessels healthier. Folic acid is commonly prescribed for people with sickle cell, especially for people with higher red blood cell production, as shown by higher counts of very young red cells (reticulocyte counts). Foods that contain high amounts of folic acid include: leafy greens such as spinach, citrus fruits, eggs, broccoli, kidney beans, and lentils.

A balanced healthy diet is a good idea for a person with sickle cell disease.

Eat plenty of fruits and vegetables along with some meat or other protein. The "heart-healthy" food choices that are high in antioxidants and omega-3 fatty acids (fish oil) are good for sickle cell disease. If you are looking for a snack, choose a fruit or vegetable instead of packaged snack foods that are sugary or fried. A handful of nuts can be a great snack too.

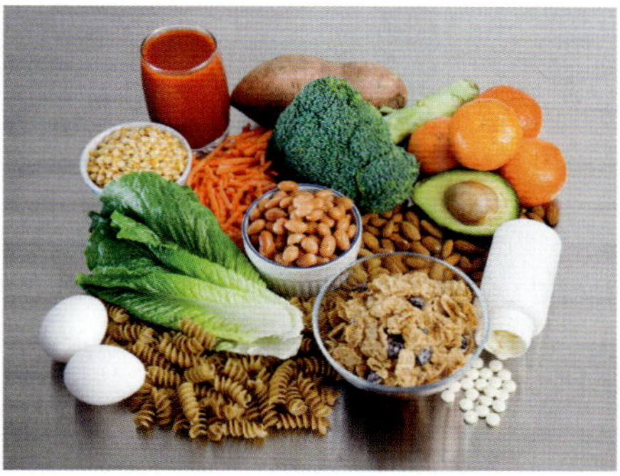

Eating foods rich in folic acid can help your body make red blood cells.

Scientists are studying whether nutritional supplements will help people with sickle cell disease. Right now, these studies have not provided solid answers.

THIRSTY?

The simple act of consuming extra water can dramatically delay the sickling effect. Even a little bit of water can make a tremendous difference. Drinking 10% more water, for example, can slow down sickling by 1,700%!

It is especially important for children with sickle cell to drink plenty of water, because kidneys—along with all other organs—are damaged by sickle cells. Once damaged, the kidneys cannot help the body retain water very well. Loss of water through urine continues at a high rate all day and all night, so it is very easy for people with sickle cell to quickly become dehydrated if they do not drink enough to replace the lost fluids.

The best fluid for children with sickle cell is water. When the sickle red blood cells get dry, they sickle. When sickle red blood cells have more water, they stay more flexible. That keeps the blood flowing better. When you drink more water, you're helping your body prevent sickle cells from getting stuck and causing pain. Other fluids like juice, milk, soup and fruit are also fine to add variation, as are popsicles. Too many sugary carbonated drinks like soda can cause cavities. Drinks with caffeine (like soda, coffee and energy drinks), alcohol, or theophylline (the specific chemical which is found in tea) make the kidney release more water into the urine. Try to limit these drinks to no more than two glasses a day.

The amount of water you need to drink depends on your size. What pediatricians call the maintenance rate of fluids is the minimum you need to avoid dehydration. The chart below indicates how much an individual child should drink. Drinking more than the amount shown is fine. Drinking even more liquids may be necessary when you are ill, exercising, or hot. When you are having sickle cell pain, make sure that you drink at least the higher of the recommended amounts.

Recommended Daily Water Consumption

Metric		**English**	
Body weight (kilograms)	Range per day (liters)	Body weight (pounds)	Range per day (8-ounce cups)
5	0.5 to 0.7	10	2 to 3
10	1.0 to 1.4	25	4 to 6
15	1.2 to 1.8	30	5 to 8
20	1.4 to 2.2	45	6 to 9
25	1.5 to 2.3	55	7 to 10
30	1.7 to 2.5	75	8 to 11
35	1.8 to 2.7	100	9 to 13
45	2.0 to 3.0	130	10 to 15
55	2.3 to 3.4	150	11 to 17
65	2.5 to 3.8	175	12 to 18
75	2.8 to 4.1		

EXERCISE? STAYING ACTIVE WITH SICKLE CELL DISEASE

Many people are mistaken in thinking that having sickle cell disease means they should avoid physical activity. This is not true! Exercise can actually encourage blood flow and help reduce crises or complications. You can stay active by choosing moderate types of exercise: yoga, walking, swimming in a heated pool, volleyball, shooting basketballs, etc. Avoid heavy joint impact like you would experience on a trampoline. Plan time to rest after exercise; rest breaks every twenty minutes are a good idea. Don't forget to drink plenty of liquids, and don't push it too hard! Listen to your body.

TREATMENTS AT HOME

One way to remember the things you can do at home to help prevent sickle cell pain problems is the word **FARMS**:

🥤 **F**luids. Drinking a lot of fluids can help prevent red blood cells from sickling.

💨 **A**ir. Get enough oxygen by taking deep breaths. Avoid conditions in which there is low oxygen, such as at high altitudes (over about 8,000 feet or about 2,500 meters). If you have asthma, be sure to treat it properly so that you do not have trouble breathing.

😴 **R**est, relaxation. Take a rest break for a few minutes if you are playing or working vigorously. Build in breaks to relax if you are having a lot of emotional stress.

💊 **M**edications, medical care. Take medicines as prescribed by your doctors. See your doctors for regular check-ups, not just when you have pain or fever, so that problems can be detected early or even prevented. Ask questions about what else you can do to help yourself take care of your sickle cell disease.

🥰 **S**ituations, support. Avoid situations that can cause problems for your sickle cell disease: avoid getting chilled by wet clothing. Pay attention to the weather forecast and bring an umbrella if rain is likely. Friends might remind you to take a bottle of water with you when you are going out to play ball.

EMERGENCY GUIDE: WHEN TO SEE THE DOCTOR

It is very important that every person or family with a young child who has sickle cell disease has a plan for how to get help immediately, at any hour, if there is a problem. Be sure to find a place that will have access to your medical records, or bring a copy that you have handy at home with you.

TIP: Use the My Health Passport on page 51 of this book, make copies of it and hang them on your refrigerator at home, so at any time when you might need it, you'll have this information handy.

Go to an emergency room or urgent care facility right away for:

* Fever above 101°F (38.5°C)
* Difficulty breathing
* Chest pain
* Abdominal (belly) swelling
* Severe headache
* Sudden weakness or loss of feeling and movement
* Seizure
* Painful erection of the penis that lasts more than four hours

Call a doctor right away for:

* Pain anywhere in the body that will not go away with treatment at home
* Any sudden problem with vision

STREET DRUGS, TOBACCO, MARIJUANA, ALCOHOL

Stay away from these substances! They are powerfully addictive. Drugs that are inhaled or smoked are damaging to your lungs, and we know that lung problems can greatly raise your chances of sickle cell pain and acute chest syndrome. Alcohol can cause your body to become dehydrated much more easily, causing the blood cells to stick together and trigger a pain episode.

VACCINATIONS

Be sure to stay current with the vaccinations that are recommended by your doctor, starting in childhood and continuing all the way through adulthood. Vaccinations are an important protection against viral infections that can become life-threatening. The American Academy of Pediatrics strongly recommends children and adults receive vaccinations and provides a schedule for immunizations at their website as well as through the Centers for Disease Control.

Beware of misinformation about vaccinations. Studies linking vaccinations to autism were withdrawn because the data was found to be faked, but they keep echoing across the Internet even though solid evidence has disproven them. Some people also continue to mistakenly believe that rare side effects of vaccines are worse than the real dangers of diseases that can be prevented by vaccines. This way of thinking has led to tragic measles cases in unvaccinated communities. Always talk to your doctor if you have questions or concerns about vaccines.

SICKLE CELL AND COVID-19

In December 2019, the World Health Organization identified, in China, a new type of virus now called COVID-19. This virus is very contagious, passed from person to person by coughing, sneezing, and touching recently contaminated surfaces, very similar to the way the common cold or flu virus is spread. This virus spread rapidly across the world in 2020, causing a global pandemic. COVID-19 caused many deaths by attacking the lungs, causing blood clots and organ failure. The Centers for Disease Control and Prevention, or CDC, has sad that people who have sickle cell disease are considered to be at increased risk for complications from COVID-19.

COVID-19 causes many of the same symptoms as the flu, nasal allergies, and the common cold. The only sure way to know is to do a home test or go to a clinic for testing. Most people who have COVID-19 experience symptoms such as fever, cough, sore throat, loss of smell or taste, nasal congestion, muscle aches, and tiredness. If you have any of these symptoms, take a home COVID test and call your doctor right away to discuss what you should do next. Call 911 for emergency care if you have difficulty breathing, unusual persistent pain or pressure in your chest, new confusion or inability to wake up easily, bluish lips or face, a severe pain episode, or increasing weakness.

What can I do to prevent getting COVID-19?

* Get vaccinated and boosted. This is the most effective step.
* Stay home as much as possible. Avoid crowds, wear a mask in public (N95 mask is best), and practice social distancing.
* Wash your hands with soap and water for 20 seconds (don't stop until

you finish singing the "alphabet song") or use hand sanitizer with at least 60% alcohol.

* Avoid touching your eyes, nose, mouth, and face.
* If you feel sick, take a test and call your medical provider immediately. Get the oral treatment Paxlovid if you are positive for COVID-19 to prevent serious complications.
* Avoid being close to people who are visibly sick, coughing, or sneezing.
* Greet others from a distance or with fist bumps (no hugs or handshakes).
* Disinfect frequently touched objects and surfaces.
* Cover your cough or sneeze with a tissue you can discard, then immediately wash your hands.

How can I be prepared?

* Please check to see if you have refilled all your medications and are not about to run out.
* Contact your doctor to ask about getting extra medications to have on hand in case there is an outbreak of COVID-19 in your community and you need to stay home for a while. Some pharmacies are offering home delivery.
* Be sure you have over-the-counter medicines to treat fever and other symptoms (e.g. Tylenol, decongestants, etc.) and medical supplies (e.g. tissues, hand sanitizers).
* Make sure you have a thermometer to take your temperature.
* Take your prescribed medications for sickle cell disease (hydroxyurea, glutamine, penicillin, folic acid, voxelotor, crizanlizumab, deferasirox, and any others). These medications will help keep your body in the best possible condition to fight off infection.
* Have enough household items and groceries on hand so that you will be prepared to stay at home for a long time.
* Find out if attending school from home is an option.

What are some good ways to stay as healthy as possible?

* Take your medications as prescribed.
* Eat a healthy diet.
* Stay hydrated.
* Try to get good rest.

I think I am having a pain crisis episode. What should I do?

Call your doctor to get advice on what to do. Consider the benefit of managing pain at home versus the risk of getting exposed to someone with COVID-19 in the clinic, emergency department, or hospital. If it feels like a typical pain crisis episode for you, they may suggest you try to do everything you can to manage your pain at home. If you are comfortable trying to manage at home, ask your doctor to call in prescriptions for pain medications. If you have symptoms of COVID-19, you should tell your doctor, "This feels different from my usual pain crisis," and ask what you should do next. Make sure you have checked your temperature because you will be asked if you did.

How do I stay informed?

Go to *OneSCDVoice.com*, SCDAA's online information superhighway where we will post updates regularly that are specific to sickle cell disease. It is free to join. We are not aware of any other more trusted resource specifically for individuals with sickle cell disease.

Go to the CDC's website (*cdc.gov/covid19*) where regularly updated information on COVID-19 will give you the latest guidelines and recommendations.

DEALING WITH THE PAIN OF SICKLE CELL DISEASE

PAIN, PAIN, GO AWAY!

Sickle cell disease can cause pain. Generally, pain affects the long bones, the spine, and the ribcage. Sometimes it is an ache that is not too bad. Sometimes the pain can be more intense and needs medicine. Sometimes the pain is really too much to handle at home and you have to go to the hospital for treatment.

One way to look at different levels of sickle cell pain is to think of stairs. Pretend that more intense pain is like being higher off the ground. Pretend that climbing higher up some stairs means reaching that level of pain with more pain treatment. We can stack up pain treatments to match the intensity of the pain.

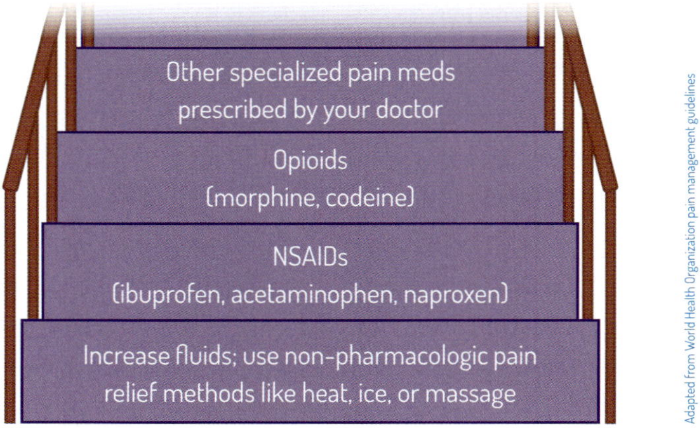

Think of your pain like stairs. Depending on your pain level, your doctors can stack different treatments to match the intensity of your pain.

WHAT CAN I DO TO PREVENT SICKLE CELL PAIN?

Unpredictable severe pain which doctors call "vaso-occlusive pain," and which is a classic symptom of sickle cell disease, sometimes can come on without any apparent reason. Some people with sickle cell disease report an early warning sensation before the pain.

Sometimes vaso-occlusive pain can be triggered by dehydration, exhaustion, infection, low oxygen, emotional stress, change of weather or chilled skin.

THINGS YOU CAN DO FOR YOURSELF TO HELP AVOID PAIN:

* Take in more fluids so that you avoid dehydration. When you notice that a trigger for pain is coming along, drink more fluids!
* Always drink more fluids when the weather changes or when the weather is very hot.
* Avoid triggers like exhaustion from too much exercise, or exhaustion from poor sleep; get enough rest.

* Avoid triggers such as getting chilled after swimming—get a towel and dry yourself quickly.
* Stay current on all vaccinations/immunizations recommended by your doctor.

A medication called hydroxyurea cannot cure sickle cell disease completely, but it can make sickle cell disease less severe and painful. Hydroxyurea works by making your red blood cells less likely to sickle so they can move through small blood vessels more easily. In 2017, a new version of hydroxyurea just for kids, called Siklos, was approved by the Food and Drug Administration, a government organization that makes sure medicines are safe and effective. Talk to your hematology doctor about whether hydroxyurea is right for you. You can read more about hydroxyurea under the medical treatment section on page 27.

Also in 2017, the FDA approved a new treatment for sickle cell disease called glutamine, and it's sold under the brand name Endari. Instead of a pill, this medication is a flavorless powder that you can mix into food or drink, and works by reducing cell damage and inflammation in the body. You can read more about glutamine under the medical treatment section on page 28.

A NEW ONLINE TOOL TO HELP WITH AT-HOME PAIN MANAGEMENT: PINPOINT™

Pinpoint™ is a new online pain assessment tool that provides a safe, convenient way for teens like you to learn about, track, evaluate, and communicate about your sickle cell pain with your medical team and parents right from your smartphone or tablet. Pinpoint™ offers an innovative Pain Assessment Tool and a Pain Diary to log physical and emotional pain symptoms. All with the touch of a finger, you can describe and assess your pain: where it hurts and for how long, how bad the pain is, and what was happening when the pain started. Pinpoint™ can send this information to your parents and your medical team via e-mail, and you can even print the report to keep in your records. Pinpoint™ is a web app and works on any smartphone or smart mobile device. You can play games, watch videos, learn preventive health tips, and visit the Patient Stories section with real stories and inspirational messages told by other sickle cell patients. Pinpoint™ also includes various relaxation activities to help you manage your pain at home. Pinpoint™ was developed by Klein Buendel, Hilton Publishing Company, and a large team of medical experts and parents of children with sickle cell disease. A research study funded by the National Institutes of Health found that Pinpoint™ was clinically proven to help teens manage their SCD pain. Pinpoint™ will be made available by subscription to patients, parents, providers and clinics in 2023 through HPC International, Inc., the parent company of Hilton Publishing Company. You can find more information on HPC's website at *www.hpcinternationalinc.com*.

OTHER EFFECTS OF SICKLE CELL DISEASE

WHY DOES SICKLE CELL DISEASE MAKE MY EYES YELLOW?

Jaundice is a sign of the breakdown of sickle red blood cells, and jaundiced eyes can be a baseline characteristic of people with sickle cell. The yellow color will be more intense as the red blood cells break down more quickly or if you do not drink enough fluids. It is not contagious, but some people become very self-conscious about jaundice. See page 70 for more discussion about jaundice.

WHY ARE SOME CHILDREN WITH SICKLE CELL DISEASE SMALLER OR SLOWER TO DEVELOP?

Having sickle cell disease can slow your growth. Children with sickle cell tend to have low weight, and bone development can be delayed. Puberty might start later for teens with sickle cell disease. It may be hard for you to

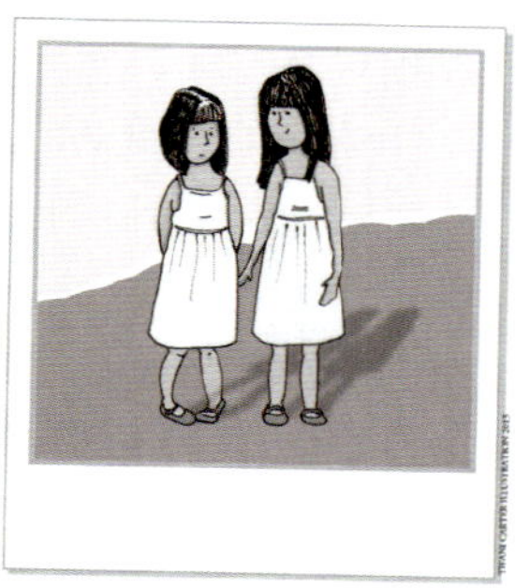

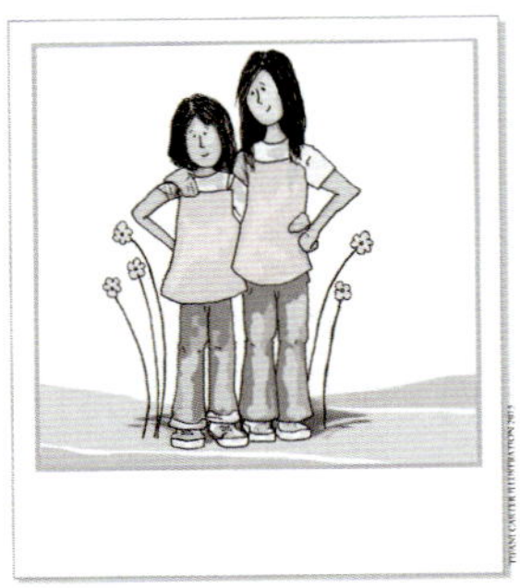

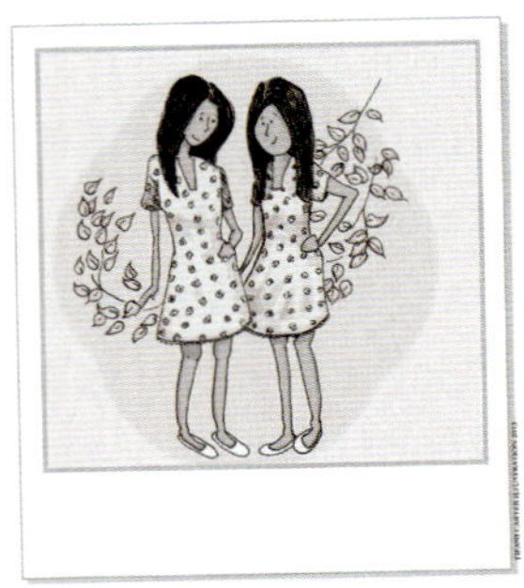

be shorter or smaller than your classmates or relatives, but you will eventually catch up and reach a typical adult height by your early twenties. In severe cases of delayed growth and development, hormonal therapy may help to reverse the problem.

Low weight has a good point—obesity is rarer in people with sickle cell disease. This may be one reason why type 2 diabetes, which is associated strongly with obesity, is relatively rare in people with sickle cell disease, even though it is quite common in people with sickle trait.

Growth can improve on anti-sickling treatments such as hydroxyurea, monthly transfusions, or a bone marrow transplant.

WHY DOES SICKLE CELL DISEASE CAUSE BED-WETTING?

Bed-wetting at night (enuresis) can be caused by the effect of sickle cell disease on the kidneys. Normally, the body sends signals to the kidneys during sleep so that the kidneys make less urine at night. This would allow you to sleep through the night with a bladder that is not very full.

STORIES FROM KIDS LIKE YOU

Spending days in the hospital is not pleasant, especially on the eve of such an important date for teenagers as my 15th birthday. This was especially true for me since I had experienced a very turbulent year with many losses. I just wanted to get well. In the week of 15th birthday, a painful crisis ended my happiness. That day everything was very simple. I was treated and released. However, my parents, always careful and concerned did not let me participate in the celebrations of my own birthday. They knew best, because two days later I was hospitalized with a high fever and diagnosed with double pneumonia. Everything that I did not want happened... It was the worst week for anyone was planning a big party for a 15th birthday. However, that week made me realize how much moments of pain makes us value happiness and who really cares for us. Nowadays, because of the care, concerns and precautions of my parents, I do not spend days in the hospital. Now I am just a visitor.

Caroline, 17 years old

Kidneys damaged by sickle cell disease cannot respond to these night-time signals to make less urine, so the kidneys make urine all through the night and fill up the bladder. If you do not wake up to use the bathroom in the middle of the night, your body can release the bladder while you are asleep, causing you to wet the bed.

Bed-wetting can be embarrassing and may hold you back from activities such as having sleepover visits with friends. This is one of the reasons that summer camp sessions specializing in children and teens with SCD are popular, allowing them to see that other children are dealing with the same problem.

Sleeping on a waterproof pad or with pull-up absorbent pants can help for a while. Most hematologists will recommend you avoid using nasal spray medicine such as desmopressin, a synthetic hormone used to reduce urine production to help minimize how frequently you must go to the bathroom, because generally a person with SCD can have kidney damage which will not respond well to the medication.

Tips for avoiding bed-wetting

* Learn what it feels like to have a full bladder and the urge to release it.
* Night-lights can make it easier for you to get to the bathroom at night.
* An alarm clock or a bed-wetting alarm on the underwear can help.
* Parents should avoid punishing bed-wetting that is associated with SCD and instead use encouragement and a reward system.

What is a bed-wetting alarm?

A bed-wetting alarm is a small machine that makes a noise or a buzzing vibration when it detects moisture. The alarm is attached to your underwear or pajamas in the area where the first drop of urine would occur when the bladder releases. The alarm goes off and alerts those in range that wetting is occurring. When you hear or feel the alarm, you'll wake up and use the bathroom. Gradually, you'll learn to respond to the feeling of a full bladder by waking and going to the bathroom before the alarm goes off. Alarm training is a type of behavioral conditioning.

MEDICAL TREATMENTS

HYDROXYUREA

What is hydroxyurea?

Hydroxyurea is a medicine that is taken daily to help make severe sickle cell disease become a milder disease. Hydroxyurea is not a treatment for pain once a pain episode has started. It is not a cure for sickle cell, but it has been used to control symptoms since the 1990s. In 2014, the National Institutes of Health stated that children as young as nine months could benefit from taking hydroxyurea, and in 2017 a new form of hydroxyurea just for kids was approved by the Food and Drug Administration.

How does it help people with sickle cell disease?

Hydroxyurea can raise your level of fetal hemoglobin and increase the size of your red blood cells—both of these effects will make the red blood cell less likely to sickle. Hydroxyurea also makes the red blood cells less sticky so that they move through small blood vessels more easily. In addition, hydroxyurea helps block some of the abnormal properties of other blood cells and blood vessels, which also helps blood flow more easily.

Hydroxyurea is helpful

Hydroxyurea usually prevents about half of a patient's problems with pain episodes and acute chest syndrome. This means fewer blood transfusions and longer periods of time between hospitalizations. People on hydroxyurea have fewer unpredictable absences from school or work, which helps them fulfill their education and career goals.

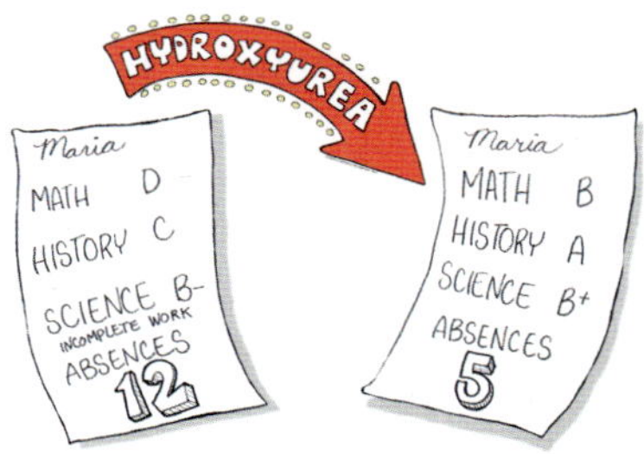
HYDROXYUREA
Maria
MATH D
HISTORY C
SCIENCE B-
INCOMPLETE WORK
ABSENCES
12
Maria
MATH B
HISTORY A
SCIENCE B+
ABSENCES
5

Hydroxyurea can also prevent some priapism, painful erections of the penis lasting longer than four hours. Sickle cell patients who take hydroxyurea tend to live longer and maintain good brain function longer, and children on hydroxyurea gain weight better.

What to check while you are on hydroxyurea

If you take hydroxyurea, you should have frequent blood tests in order to monitor your blood counts. Taking hydroxyurea might cause a risk to a fetus if the mother or father is taking hydroxyurea at the time of conception, so an acceptable method of birth control is necessary while taking hydroxyurea.

GLUTAMINE

L-glutamine oral powder is a new prescription medication for sickle cell disease. It was approved by the FDA in 2017 and first entered the US market in 2018 under the brand name Endari®.

How does glutamine work?

Glutamine is an amino acid. It is part of the food protein that we eat. Glutamine works primarily by boosting the antioxidant properties of the red blood cell. Antioxidants help the body minimize oxidant damage. Oxidant damage is the same thing that causes iron to rust and sliced apples and avocados to turn brown, and in the human body it increases the risk of cancer, heart disease, and stroke. Sickled red cells have more oxidant damage than other red cells. By boosting the antioxidant properties in red blood cells, glutamine helps the body fight oxidant damage and cut down on inflammation.

What are the benefits of glutamine?

Glutamine may help make sickle cell disease milder. Research shows that people taking glutamine had fewer pain episodes, spent less time in the hospital, and had acute chest syndrome less often. Glutamine does not cure sickle cell disease.

Glutamine appears to be safe, and only one out of ten people participating in trials prior to FDA approval had any side effects at all. The side effects that were reported include constipation, gurgle noises from the stomach, nausea, and chest tightness. Regular blood tests to monitor organ functions are not needed for patients on glutamine.

How do I take glutamine?

Glutamine that is used as medication has been purified and comes in packets of powder, each about half the size of a packet of hot chocolate mix. Stir the powder in a drink or food like water, juice, milk, applesauce, or yogurt. Glutamine is usually taken twice a day, but be sure to take the number of packets prescribed by your doctor as directed.

NEWLY APPROVED TREATMENTS

In 2019, the FDA approved two new treatments for sickle cell disease: voxelotor and crizanlizumab.

Voxelotor is sold under the brand name Oxbryta® and it's for everyone age four and up. It's a pill you take once a day, and it can help increase your hemoglobin levels while decreasing the destruction of red blood cells (hemolysis). Some research is showing that voxelotor can even make your red blood cells more flexible, which helps your blood flow better.

Crizanlizumab-tmca is sold under the brand name Adakveo® and you can take it starting at age sixteen. It's given through an IV once a month and can help reduce pain crises.

BLOOD TRANSFUSION

Many problems with sickle cell disease can be managed through blood transfusions.

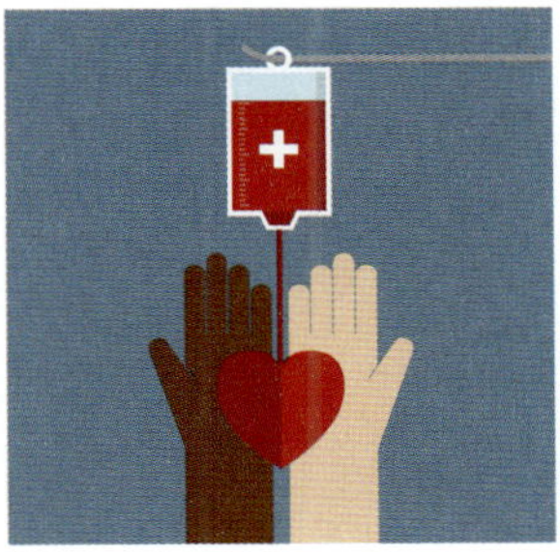

iStock / Getty Images

What is a blood transfusion? How is it done?

A blood transfusion is a safe, common procedure in which you receive blood through an intravenous (IV) line inserted into one of your blood vessels. Through this line, you receive red blood cells that do not sickle.

A nurse will bring in a bag of blood that has been specially selected for you. The bag will hang on a pole near your hospital bed and a tube will be inserted into the bag. Then the blood can travel from the bag, through the IV and into your blood vessels. The procedure usually takes one to four hours, depending on how much blood you need.

Most of the time, you will not feel any discomfort when the blood goes in. Nurses and others will make sure you feel okay during the transfusion. A nurse keeps an eye on your temperature and blood pressure and looks to make sure there is no rash or other signs of an allergic reaction.

When does a person with sickle cell get a transfusion?

A transfusion can provide improved oxygen flow for a short time when anemia is very severe or when your body is going through severe stress. These are some of the sickle cell problems that might require a transfusion:

* aplastic crisis
* acute spleen problems
* acute chest syndrome
* severe illness
* preparation for surgery or general anesthesia

Some patients get transfusions every month for years to reduce the effects of sickle red blood cells. Regular transfusions might also be used if there are long-term problems with major organs like the heart, lungs or kidneys. An abnormal result from an ultrasound test called a transcranial Doppler scan can also make regular transfusions necessary in an effort to prevent a stroke.

What is "simple transfusion" or "top-off transfusion"?

Simple transfusions can be used for short problems that go away in a few days or weeks. A simple transfusion might provide one to three units of donor red blood cells, which will raise your hemoglobin level so that you become less anemic. Sometimes a simple transfusion is called a "top-off transfusion" because it is like filling a gas tank.

Monthly simple transfusions can be repeated every two to four weeks to keep a high level of normal red blood cells for years. Your doctor will order regular blood tests to make sure that you receive the right amount of transfusion each time.

What is an exchange transfusion?

An exchange transfusion means that red blood cells are removed from the body at the same time that new red blood cells are transfused into the patient. This type of transfusion is used to rapidly replace sickle cells with normal cells. A machine can perform exchange transfusion quickly and safely in a process called automated erythrocytapheresis. The major concerns with this procedure include increased red cell utilization (twice as many blood units might be used for each exchange transfusion compared to a simple transfusion), venous access (you'll need to have good veins that can take large needles for the exchange transfusion), and increased cost. The major plus with erythrocytapheresis is its success in decreasing iron overload burden.

How is my blood matched?

Before you get a blood transfusion, you will need to give a small blood sample. Why? So your blood can be tested to determine your blood type in order to find the best match for you from the blood bank.

Special notes about transfusions

* Relatives should not be used as blood donors for children who could be candidates for bone marrow transplantation.
* Autologous blood transfusions (transfusions using blood you have donated yourself) for patients with sickle cell disease should be avoided.
* Red cell substitutes are experimental and generally not useful for sickle cell problems.

What is blood type? What is blood phenotype?

Red blood cells have many variations in the pattern of their surface molecules (**antigens**). Many people know the most famous antigens: blood types A, B, O and AB, and Rh positive or negative. There are many other blood antigens with names like Fy, Jk, Kell, and S, which are known to blood specialists.

The **blood phenotype** is the pattern of all surface molecules. Your phenotype pattern is recognized by your immune system like the pattern of a fingerprint or the pattern of an electronic bar code.

If the donor blood is not closely matched to your own blood, your body may build antibodies against the donated blood and the transfusions will be ineffective in treating the symptoms of the disease. Like other genetic factors, blood is similar among people of the same ethnic group, which is why the closest match for an African-American sickle cell patient will most likely come from an African-American donor.

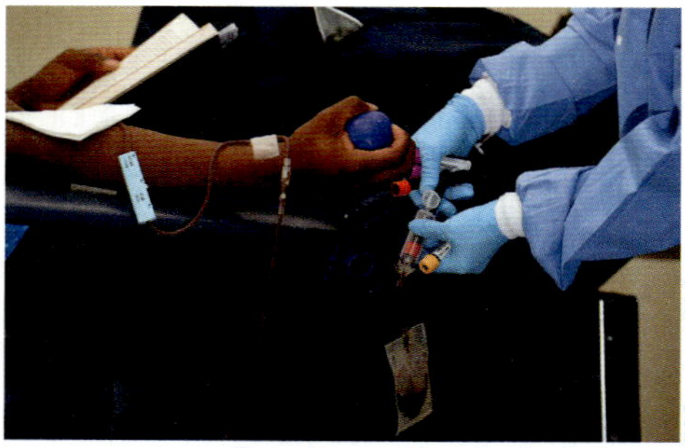

U.S. Department of Defense

The closest blood match for an African-American recipient is usually an African-American donor.

When your immune system "examines" the phenotype of the red blood cells coming in from the donor, sometimes the immune system will attack the transfused donor cells because the phenotype of the donor is too different from the phenotype of the recipient. The immune system then makes antibodies that recognize the donor cells and tag them for destruction. This immune attack is called hemolytic transfusion reaction and is very dangerous for the recipient of a blood transfusion. In a hemolytic transfusion reaction, antibodies bind a group of chemicals called complement to the surface of the donor red cell, punching holes through the surface and breaking the cell open. This destruction of the red blood cell is called hemolysis. Sometimes, antibodies make the special cells of the spleen or liver trap the donor red cells and pull them out of the circulation, then engulf them and destroy them more like an amoeba eating a germ.

The best way to reduce the risk of hemolytic transfusion reaction is to match the phenotypes of the donor and the recipient as closely as possible. The blood bank knows the blood phenotypes of people who receive monthly transfusions and looks for donors who are close to the same phenotype. Some blood banks call these donors the "blood buddies" of the recipient.

What does the blood donor lose?

The person who donates blood gives up about a pint, or 400 to 600 mL of blood. Drinking water, juice and other fluids can replace the fluid lost within an hour. However, every blood donor also gives up a little iron from the body. People who donate blood regularly should eat foods that are rich in iron. A well-balanced diet will restore the iron in about one month. Eating foods that provide plenty of vitamin C together with iron-rich foods will help the body absorb iron better. On the other hand, drinking tea and other caffeinated drinks will interfere with iron absorption. It is safe and no big deal for a healthy person to donate a small amount of blood. Your mom or dad might have done this. Kids don't usually donate blood, but it is a good thing to do when you are older.

What does the blood donor gain?

Blood donors are often volunteers and they do not get paid. But they might get some refreshments from the donor center to help rebuild their blood, and, more importantly, they get the satisfaction of helping others in need.

What is a blood bank?

In poorer countries, donors are often relatives or friends of the person who needs a transfusion. The donation is made just before the blood is transfused. In the United States and many other countries, groups of healthy volunteers give their blood for people who they might never meet. The blood is stored in plastic bags and usually frozen.

Healthy, donated blood is very valuable stuff. They even call the place that collects it the blood BANK. Get it? A bank is a safe place for money and other valuables.[1]

What problems can occur with a blood transfusion?

Each year, almost 5 million Americans will need a blood transfusion. Most transfusions go well, but mild complications can occur. Very rarely, serious problems develop.

---

1 *https://kidshealth.org/en/teens/transfusions.html*

Transfusion reactions. There are several types of reactions, and some are worse than others. Some reactions happen as soon as the transfusion is started, while others take several days or even longer to develop. Many precautions are taken before a transfusion is started in order to keep reactions from happening. The blood type of the unit is checked many times, and the unit is cross-matched to be sure that it matches the blood type of the person who will get it. After that, both a nurse and a blood bank lab technician look at the information about the patient and the information on the unit of blood (or blood component) before it is released. The information is double-checked once more in the patient's presence before the transfusion is started.

Infected blood unit. Blood transfusions can transmit infections caused by bacteria, viruses and parasites. Infections from blood transfusions have become extremely rare with careful testing and donor screening. If a blood unit passes through these steps, the chance that it is infected is estimated to be 1 in 650,000. People who have certain illnesses such as hepatitis or HIV are not allowed to donate blood because they could pass their sickness on to another person through a blood transfusion. After blood is collected, blood banks test it very carefully to make sure the blood is free of diseases and germs. The blood bank discards any blood that could make someone sick.

Allergic reaction. Hives (an itchy swollen rash) can be the signal of an allergic reaction. These can be treated with antihistamine medication before the reaction gets worse. Allergic reactions during a transfusion usually occur because of the body's reaction to plasma proteins in the donated blood.

Fever. A sudden fever during a transfusion or within twenty-four hours after a transfusion can be the body's response to white blood cells in the transfusion. People who have had a fever reaction are usually given blood units that are leukoreduced. This means that the white blood cells have been removed from the donor blood by filters or other means,[2] which can

---

2 *https://www.cancer.org/treatment/treatments-and-side-effects/treatment-types/blood-transfusion-and-donation/how-blood-transfusions-are-done.html*

reduce the occurrence of complications or side effects from receiving multiple transfusions.

Acute immune hemolytic reaction. This is the most serious type of transfusion reaction and it is very rare. It happens when donor and patient blood types do not match. The patient's antibodies attack the transfused red blood cells, causing them to break open (hemolyze) and release harmful substances into the bloodstream. Patients may have chills, fever, chest and lower back pain, and nausea. The kidneys may be badly damaged and dialysis may be needed. A hemolytic reaction can be deadly if the transfusion is not stopped as soon as the reaction starts.

Delayed hemolytic reaction. This type of reaction happens when the body slowly attacks antigens (other than ABO antigens) on the transfused blood cells. The blood cells are broken down days or weeks after the transfusion. There are usually no symptoms, but the transfused red blood cells are destroyed and the patient's red blood cell count falls. In rare cases, the kidneys may be affected and treatment may be needed. One way this might show up is through brown urine that is the color of cola. People do not usually have this type of reaction unless they have had transfusions in the past. If you do have this type of reaction, you'll need special blood testing before any more blood can be transfused. Units of blood that do not have the antigen that the body is attacking must be used.

Iron overload. Each transfusion of red blood cells adds a little iron to the body. Repeated monthly transfusions will probably result in iron overload. The body can run out of places to store the iron, and iron could end up with too much iron in places like the heart, liver and glands. This excess iron can lead to serious damage to the body and needs to be treated with a group of medications called "chelators." The chelators help the body to excrete iron.

adapted from http://www.redcrossblood.org

CURING SICKLE CELL DISEASE

Cures for sickle cell disease by transplant of bone marrow or stem cells have been successful since the mid-1990s (more than 1,600 people cured by transplant at the time of this writing). Transplant is making rapid progress although it is not yet ready for every person with sickle cell disease. You should talk to your doctor and your parents regularly about new information available for sickle cell patients. Lots of doctors, nurses and scientists are working hard every day to find new ways to treat and cure sickle cell disease.

BONE MARROW TRANSPLANTATION

What is bone marrow?

The soft spongy stuff in the middle of bones is called bone marrow. Marrow contains blood stem cells, which produce the cells of the blood: red blood cells that carry oxygen, white blood cells that fight infection and platelets that stop bleeding. Some people call the marrow the "blood factory."

BONE MARROW TRANSPLANT DONOR

Who may be a good match?

- Brothers and sisters: 25% chance of identical HLA

Other relatives?

- Parents: "haploidentical" half-match
- Grandpa, aunt, cousin: unlikely to match

Exception: closely inbred clans

What is the connection between bone marrow and sickle cell disease?

Sickle genes tell the bone marrow stem cells to make abnormal red blood cells that contain sickle hemoglobin instead of normal hemoglobin. It makes sense that to cure sickle cell requires correction of the bone marrow stem cells.

Finding a bone marrow donor who does not have sickle cell trait or a sickle cell gene at all means that donor's marrow stem cells can make healthy, normal red blood cells that will not sickle.

How is the bone marrow donated? Is it surgery?[3]

It is surgery, but not with a scalpel. Marrow cells are collected from the pelvic bone (between the spine and where a hip pocket would be) using a special needle. Donors receive general anesthesia so no pain is experienced during the marrow extraction, which takes about two hours. The donor ends up with large bandage on the area. Within a week of donating, most donors can to return to work, school and many regular activities. The donor's marrow grows back within a few weeks.

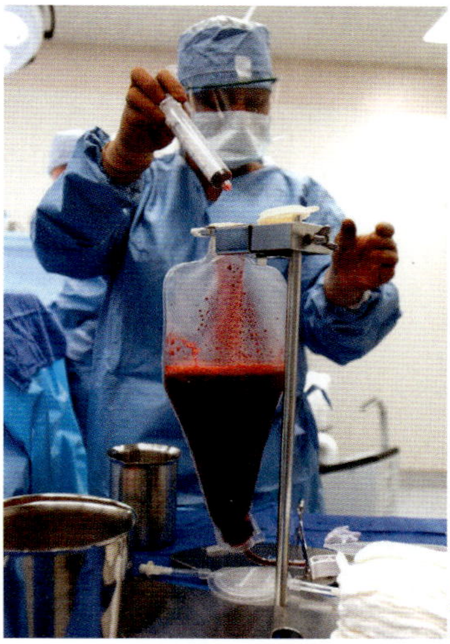

U.S. Navy

After bone marrow is collected, it's placed into a sterile bag in preparation for transfusion into the recipient.

Are blood stem cells only found in the bone marrow?

Some stem cells are also found in the blood, especially in a newborn baby's blood. These stem cells can also be used for transplants.

The placenta and umbilical cord are attached to the baby in the womb, but they are then set aside after the baby is born. Cord blood can be collected from the placenta and umbilical cord after birth without any harm to the baby.

Blood stem cells are also present in small quantities in the blood of an adult. Donors receive daily injections of a medicine called filgrastim for four days before and on the first day of the collection to increase the number of stem cells in the bloodstream. The blood stem cells can be removed by running the adult donor's blood through a filtering machine. The remaining blood flows back into the donor. The donor's blood stem cells will grow back.

---

3 Adapted from *https://www.dkms.org/donor-info/stem-cell-donation/bone-marrow-donation*

Do you know that people talk about marrow and blood like they talk about fruit trees? The cells that produce these blood cells are called "stem cells" because they are like the stem of a plant.

Fruit tree		Marrow and blood
the stem	⟷	marrow cells
leaves, flowers, and fruit	⟷	red blood cells, white blood cells, and platelets
the stem grows leaves, flowers, and fruit	⟷	marrow stem cells produce red blood cells, white blood cells, and platelets
the stem can be grafted onto another plant and will grow the leaves, flowers, and fruit that belong with that stem	⟷	marrow stem cells can be transplanted into another person and will still produce the red blood cells, white blood cells, and platelets that belong with that marrow

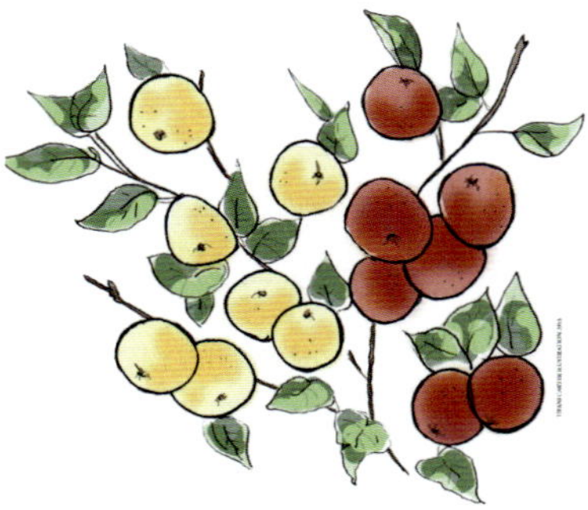

How do the stem cells get into the recipient? Is it surgery?

Bone marrow transplant is not surgery. The blood stem cells are put in a bag that looks a lot like a blood transfusion bag. The cells go through an intravenous line into the transplant recipient, just like a blood transfusion. The stem cells find their way to the bone marrow space and start to grow there.

What does HLA mean?

Human leukocyte antigen (HLA) typing is used to match patients and donors for blood stem cell transplants. HLA are proteins, or markers, found on most cells in your body. Your immune system uses these markers to recognize which cells belong in your body and which do not.

If you need a transplant, your doctor will take a blood sample to test for your HLA type. A close match between your HLA markers and your donor's can reduce the risk that your immune cells will attack your donor's cells (graft rejection) or that your donor's immune cells will attack your body after the transplant (graft versus host disease, or GVHD).

It makes sense that to cure sickle cell requires change in the bone marrow stem cells. There are three ways to do this:

* The **full**, or **myeloablative**, method uses high doses of chemotherapy to completely ablate, or wipe out, the bone marrow of the recipient. The donor blood stem cells then come in and grow over several weeks. The success rate of curing sickle cell disease with this method is about 90%. Worldwide, this approach has been done in at least 300 children. The downsides are: (1) high doses of chemo may not be tolerated by older children or adults, or those who are very ill; (2) there is a 10-20% chance of GVHD and a small proportion of patients can die of GVHD; and (3) inability to have children later.
* The **reduced-intensity** approach uses about 80% of the chemo dose of the full approach. It has the same limitation as the full approach, but the experience has been reported in twenty-nine patients at the time of this publication. The early successes need to be confirmed.
* The **non-ablative** approach uses different chemo or 30–50% of the full radiation dose. It has the advantages of safety (especially for patients who are very ill because of many problems and side effects already caused by SCD), little or no GVHD, and preservation of fertility (the ability to have children one day). The limitation of this approach is that there has been less experience with it, both in the number of patients who have tried it and the limited period of long-term follow-up since this is a newer approach. When dozens of people have had transplants with this approach, then we can see whether the transplant will last a long time and whether rare or unexpected new problems will show up. At the time of this writing, only thirty-four patients have had transplant with

this technique, and most of them are less than five years from the time of transplant. The early successes need to be confirmed.

How successful is bone marrow transplantation for sickle cell disease?
Bone marrow transplantation is mostly performed on children severely affected by sickle cell disease with donors who are an HLA-matched brother or sister. The first few transplants of this type were done in the early 1990s and had some problems, but doctors have adjusted the transplant procedures to make a special package for sickle cell patients. Since about the year 2000, these transplants have had success rates of more than 95% for children with a donor who is an HLA-matched brother or sister. As of 2018, more than 1,600 sickle cell patients have been cured through bone marrow transplantation.

CURE BY TRANSPLANTATION
Transplants from the 2000s

- 96% survival
- 93% cure of SCD

Marrow or cord blood from HLA-matched sibling is no longer experimental and is covered by insurance.

There is some chance of graft rejection, which means that you have a transplant but it is not successful in curing your sickle cell disease. There is also some chance of death.

Researchers are currently experimenting with bone marrow transplantation using donors that are not a complete HLA-match. This type of transplantation carries greater risk of complications like GVDH, but it would allow parents to be donors for their children instead of just HLA-matched siblings.

How much of the sickle cell disease will be cured by transplant?
Anemia and jaundice should go away, and there should be no new problems with pain, acute chest syndrome, priapism, spleen or other acute pain. Long-term pain might take six months or more to go away. Growth and development will probably improve, and no new strokes should occur.

However, organs already damaged by sickle cell disease will probably not heal completely. Weakness or other loss of function from previous strokes or hip damage (avascular necrosis) will not go away, but damage to kidneys or lungs might improve. In rare cases, the spleen grows back after transplant.

What are the side effects of the transplant?
Side effects of bone marrow transplants depend on the type of preparation used for the transplant. The strong chemotherapy medicines used in some transplants can make it difficult for patients to go through puberty or eventually have children. Their hair probably will fall out, but it usually will grow back. Chemotherapy can temporarily cause vomiting, but there are good medicines to control it. Infection or organ damage can cause death.

Radiation therapy can have similar effects to chemotherapy. Immunosuppressant therapy has different side effects, mainly causing the body to be wide-open to infections.

With any type of transplant, GVHD can occur. GVHD is sometimes a mild and treatable condition, but it can also become a long-term problem that might be worse than sickle cell disease in some people. GVHD can also cause death.

There is a higher risk of bad side effects if a patient was in very poor health before the transplant. To check for side effects, transplant doctors usually

A SURVIVOR'S STORY
Elvis Silva Magalhães had sickle cell disease in Brazil. He lived with frequent pain and recurrent priapism. He also had leg ulcers. He recalls many sleepless nights because of sickle cell pain. When he was 38, his brother donated bone marrow for a transplant. This made him one of the oldest people with sickle cell to have a BMT. He has been going around the country telling people about sickle cell disease.

Today he is nearly 60 years old and doing well 25 years after his bone marrow transplant. Elvis said, "I never knew I could feel this good to live without sickle cell pain." His only medication is daily penicillin because of his functional asplenia. He is among the leaders of ABRADFAL, the Brazilian advocacy group for sickle cell disease. He stands up in international meetings to speak up for more services for sickle cell. (*African Sickle Cell News & World Report* Vol. 4 (1) Jan-Mar 2012) will schedule a lot of follow-up appointments.

The newest transplant method for sickle cell is the non-ablative approach. It is also called *partial mixed chimerism*. With this method, enough donor marrow is transplanted to the patient to produce normal red blood cells. The better red blood cells produced by the donor marrow have a longer lifespan than sickle red blood cells, which will allow the healthy cells to eventually become the majority of the circulating red blood cells.

It is believed that we do not need to wipe out all of the marrow cells to put in the blood stem cells from a sibling to correct sickle cell disease. When less than full doses of chemo or radiation are used for transplant, the end result is often a mixture of patient and donor stem cells in the bone marrow. This mixture of stem cells then makes the mixture of blood cells circulating throughout the body.

Cord blood transplant

In addition to bone marrow, blood from the umbilical cord and placenta can be another source of cells for transplant. Many cord blood banks offer help with the costs of storing cord blood for a baby whose brother or sister has a disease that could be cured by cord blood transplant. Parents should inquire about sibling directed donation programs or related donor programs. A helpful guide can be found at *parentsguidecordblood.org*. Mothers who want to save their babies' cord blood should be sure that their obstetricians know before delivery that cord blood collection is desired.

Frequently asked questions about transplant

Comments from a panel discussion in Washington, DC, October 2009:

Can you participate in sports?

"I previously had a hard time running a mile; now I play field hockey."

—A high school girl cured of sickle cell, now doing well.

A young girl with sickle cell disease will have a myeloablative transplant that probably means she will not be able to have children. How do the parents make that kind of a decision?

"You take the choice for a young girl that the transplant process might cause infertility, and we decided it was better for her to survive without sickle cell disease and then adopt a child later, rather than probably die early of sickle cell problems and never be able to have children at all."

The decision to go to transplant is a very serious one, and sometimes the transplant does not go well.

"The decision for transplant is not easy, you need to ask enough questions to then be able to say 'no regrets, we would do it again.'"

—Mother of a teen who died suddenly about 3 months after a seemingly successful transplant.

GENE THERAPY

Another type of treatment that is showing great promise is gene therapy. To understand gene therapy, it helps to know about the genetic code. Every cell in your body contains DNA, which is a collection of molecules in a long chain. DNA contains the genetic code, or instructions, for the body's cells to make proteins. Think of the genetic code like a recipe for a cake—you add specific ingredients with specific measurements and follow the instructions for baking. Changes to the genetic code are responsible for mutations that can cause human disease. If you bake a cake by following a recipe that has mistakes in it, it may not taste very good—maybe you put in a whole cup of salt instead of just a teaspoon, or you bake it for only five minutes instead of twenty-five. When that happens, the cake is not going to turn out the way it's supposed to. A mutation in a person's DNA can change the way the body produces certain proteins such as hemoglobin S, the protein in red blood cells that allows blood to carry oxygen throughout the body. One goal of gene therapy is to correct DNA mutations, allowing the patient's body to produce proteins correctly and essentially curing the patient's condition.

There are different ways to treat a disease with gene therapy. The most common

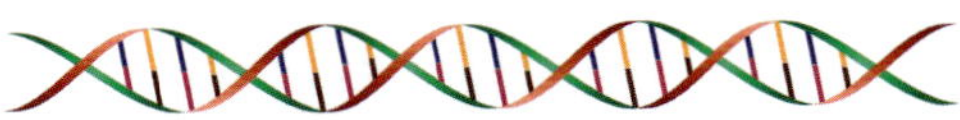

DNA is a collection of molecules in a long chain. These molecules make up the instructions for the different proteins your body needs to make.

method is to add a new, healthy gene at a random location within the patient's DNA to allow the patient's body to create normal proteins. This is most often done by taking a virus, clearing out the material that causes someone to get sick, and replacing it with a healthy gene. When the virus is introduced to the body and tries to infect healthy cells, instead of causing an illness, it inserts the healthy gene into the cell. The cell with the new gene will grow and divide, creating other cells with the healthy gene, and eventually there will be more cells with the healthy gene than with the defective gene that causes disorders like sickle cell.

Even though research is still in progress on gene therapy, there have been some promising results with viral transfer. In 2017, there was a report that researchers successfully cured a fifteen-year-old French boy of sickle cell by using gene therapy. In this boy's case, doctors used a virus to introduce DNA with the correct instructions to make healthy hemoglobin. Over time, his bone marrow began to make more and more healthy red blood cells, and fewer and fewer blood cells with sickle hemoglobin, until finally he was cured of sickle cell disease, becoming the first person in the world to be cured of SCD with gene therapy. At the time of this writing, about thirty people with SCD have been treated with viral transfer gene therapy, though it's too early to tell whether it has been successful.

A newer method of gene therapy is called gene editing, which allows genes to be added, deleted, or changed at specific points in your DNA. A clinical research study using gene editing to treat SCD began in 2019. Watch for news and studies about gene editing techniques like CRISPR, zinc fingers, and TALEN.

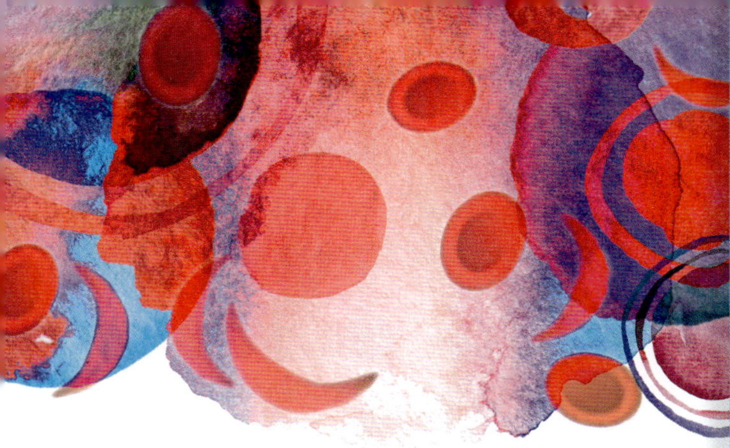

> It's important for me to keep my teachers informed. It makes it easier when I need visits to the nurse's office.
>
> —Ania, teen with SCD

SECTION 3

GROWING UP WITH Sickle Cell Disease

SCHOOL ACCOMMODATIONS

It will be helpful for your teachers and school staff to understand that you may occasionally experience pain at school. They should know that serious, often unexpected pain can be triggered by dehydration, exhaustion, infection, low oxygen, emotional stress, or change of weather.

Your teachers should know that you could become dehydrated quickly if you are not allowed to have ready access to water, either from a water bottle at your desk or from a nearby water fountain. Your teachers also need to be aware that you will need to visit the restroom more often—urination is more frequent than normal due to poor kidney function, which can begin as early as the preschool years.

Jaundiced eyes can be a baseline characteristic of people with sickle cell. It is not contagious, but some children can become very self-conscious of this.

WHAT CAN I TELL MY TEACHERS AND OTHER SCHOOL STAFF MEMBERS SO THAT THEY CAN HELP ME TO STAY WELL?

You and your family can tell your school many things about sickle cell disease:

1. **Sickle cell disease** is an inherited disorder of the blood. It is a lifelong condition that can be treated, but it has no cure except bone marrow transplantation. It is not contagious.

2. **Sickle cell disease** can cause some medical emergencies as well as hidden daily problems. However, the challenges of sickle cell disease can be very different for any two students.

3. **Physical activity**—The low red blood cell counts (anemia) of sickle cell disease can cause decreases in endurance.

   * Teachers should encourage your participation in physical education but allow rest breaks if you feel pain, shortness of breath, or weakness.
   * Some students may have bone pain or bone damage that impairs mobility, so they may have difficulty moving quickly between classrooms or on stairs.
   * It may be helpful for your school to provide an extra set of textbooks for you to keep at home in order to decrease the physical stress of carrying a heavy backpack.

4. **Fluids**—Silent kidney damage increases both urination and the chances of dehydration. Dehydration can lead to increased sickling of red blood cells and vaso-occlusive pain.

   * Your teachers should encourage you to drink plenty of fluids throughout the day. Doctors recommend allowing you to carry a water bottle with you. Going to the water fountain or cooler is also fine.
   * You should be allowed bathroom breaks whenever necessary.

5. **Temperature**—Extremely hot or cold temperatures can trigger a painful episode.

   * You should limit outdoor activities when the weather is excessively hot or cold.
   * Be sure that you dress right for the weather (including fire drills). Dressing in layers permits flexibility when weather conditions change.

* Take care to avoid excessive chilling from air conditioning or wet clothing.
* Request bus transport when it is too hot or cold to walk to school.

6. **Physical appearance**—Most people with sickle cell disease look like other typical kids.
    * Jaundice (yellow eyes) can be caused by the products of increased broken red blood cells.
    * Delayed growth and puberty appear to be caused by chronic anemia and organ damage.

WHAT CONDITIONS REQUIRE URGENT MEDICAL ATTENTION?

Vaso-occlusive pain

Unpredictable severe pain is the hallmark of sickle cell disease. Pain can be triggered and worsened by dehydration, fever, illness, and extreme hot or cold temperatures.

Pain management begins with fluids, rest and warmth. Medications may start with ibuprofen and progress to stronger oral medications. Unrelieved pain must be evaluated in the hematology clinic or the emergency department.

Fever

A temperature of 101.3° F (38.5° C) means going to the hospital right away for a medical evaluation. Due to impaired spleen function in sickle cell patients, sepsis (a bacterial blood infection) may be life-threatening within a few hours. Your family should be contacted immediately.

Other urgent conditions

Other potential emergency conditions include stroke. Your family should be contacted immediately and you should be brought to a medical facility (a hematology clinic during clinic hours or the emergency department) for a prompt medical evaluation if you experience lethargy, pallor, poor appetite, severe headache, shortness of breath or blurry vision.

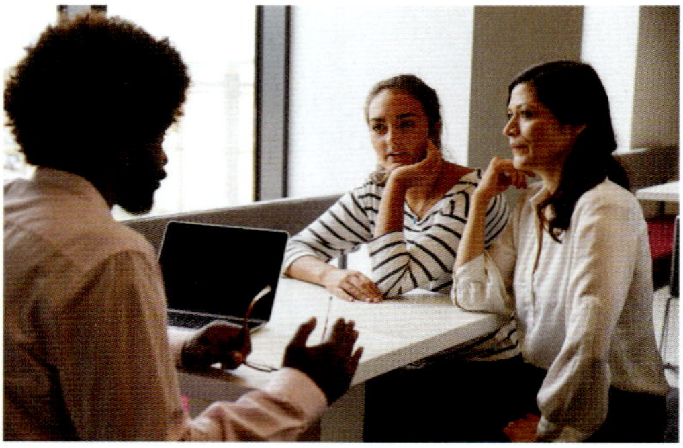

Tell your parent or guardian if you're having trouble at school and what changes might help you with your education. Meeting with your teachers or school administrators is the first step in getting the help you need.

WHAT ARE OTHER IMPLICATIONS FOR EDUCATIONAL PLANNING?

Some students need special arrangements and accommodations at school, such as an individualized educational plan (IEP), a 504 plan, and maybe tutoring.

At some point during your education, you may need to be hospitalized and miss school. You might be in the hospital for a few days for pain management or longer if other problems come up. After you are discharged, you may miss a few additional days of school to manage pain at home.

Give your teacher and school nurse the telephone numbers for your doctors and a copy of your health passport (see page 51 for a copy you can fill out, and review it with your doctor to be sure it is correct). By doing this, you can be sure that they have your most recent medical information ready in case you have any complications or issues while you are at school. You can also share these websites about sickle cell with your teachers:

* *https://www.cdc.gov/ncbddd/sicklecell/documents/tipsheet_Supporting_Students_with_SCD.pdf*
* *www.cdc.gov/ncbddd/sicklecell/documents/SCD%20factsheet_9steps.pdf*

WHY SHOULD I KEEP TRACK OF MY MEDICAL RECORDS? HOW DO I DO IT?

Every time you see your doctors or go to the hospital, they keep detailed notes in writing or on computers about your health history—these are your medical records. Doctors look up your records to remember what happened to you in the past so that they can understand better how to treat you today.

WHAT IS AN INDIVIDUALIZED EDUCATION PROGRAM (IEP)?

An IEP is a formal plan for students with disabilities to help them succeed at school through special education. The rules for creating an IEP fall under the Individuals with Disabilities Education Act, a federal law that protects children with disabilities. An IEP details your learning goals and the services your school will provide to help you reach those goals, such as how and what you learn and changes to your learning environment. To start the process of getting an IEP, your parent or guardian should contact your school principal to ask for an evaluation. Your IEP is monitored by a team that includes your parent or guardian, general and special education teachers, a school psychologist, and a school district representative who oversees special education services. Your IEP team will review your plan at least once a year, and all services will be provided for free by your school district.

WHAT IS A 504 PLAN?

A 504 plan maps out services and accommodations a school will provide to a student who has a disability but does not need special education services. Accommodations in a 504 plan might include allowing you to take extra bathroom breaks or keep a water bottle at your desk. To start the process of getting a 504 plan, your parent or guardian should contact your school to find out who the school's 504 coordinator is and ask for an evaluation. The rules for creating a 504 plan are less strict than those for an IEP, but a 504 is usually created and monitored by your parent or guardian, your teachers, and your principal or another school administrator. Your 504 plan is usually reviewed once a year, but it depends on the state you live in. Any services outlined in your 504 plan will be provided for free by your school district.

Your family probably has been keeping track of your medical records since you were born.

Many families choose one or more of these options:

* Keep copies of all medical records in a notebook or folder.
* Write notes in a notebook and bring it to all medical appointments.
* Keep a copy of just the most important papers that summarize your medical history.
* Memorize the most important information in your medical history.

All of your medical records will stay together as long as you keep going to the same doctor and hospital. When you go to a new doctor or hospital, one of the first things you will be asked is to remember all of your medical history until they can get a copy of the medical records from your other doctor or hospital. Check whether your hospital's electronic medical record system has a feature like Patient Portal or MyChart, which can allow you to access your records easily.

You can offer to help track your medical records as you grow older. When you become an adult, you will be expected to keep track of your own medical records.

Another time that you might need to have your medical records is when you travel—to camp, on a long field trip, or other trips. For this reason, a medical summary is sometimes nicknamed a health passport because it is an important set of papers, just like a passport is an important document to prove your citizenship when you travel. An example of a health passport is on the following page.

STORIES FROM KIDS LIKE YOU

My name is Samara Cristina. A few days after my birth I started getting sick with fever and infection. I started taking antibiotics and every ten days the antibiotics were changed. For months my mom and I suffered because we did not know what I had. Because my mother did not know what I had, nothing was resolved. Finally she talked to my dad, and they decided to pay for a private doctor to find out what I really had. When my mother took me to the private doctor, he asked us to take some tests. I did them. When I went back to the doctor he said that I had sickle cell anemia and explained what this was to my mother. The doctor explained that he was already suspicious that it was this disease since I was anemic, and he had already treated a boy with the same symptoms. I started the treatments when I was one year and two months old. When I was seven, my mother told me what I had. It was sickle cell anemia, and she said that I could lead a normal life, but I would have limitations. Today I'm 18 years old. I have finished my studies and I plan to go to college.

MY HEALTH PASSPORT

Name:	Date completed:
Birthdate:	Date reviewed:
Address:	Date reviewed:

SICKLE CELL HISTORY (ASK YOUR DOCTOR TO CIRCLE WHAT YOU HAVE HAD)

Sickle cell type:	SS	SC	S-beta 0-thal		S-beta plus-thal	Other
Baseline hemoglobin level:		7	8	9	10	11	12

Acute chest syndrome	Monthly transfusion	Splenic sequestration
Frequent pain	Retina problems	Gallstones casing pain
Bacteria in the blood (sepsis)	Bone infection (osteomyelitis)	Delay in growth or puberty
Priapism	Hip damage (avascular necrosis)	Stroke
Weakness of arm	Weakness of leg	Difficulty with reading
Difficulty with memory	Difficulty with organizing	

OTHER KEY HISTORY

RBC alloantibodies	Central venous line	Port under the skin

Hospitals where I have been transfused:

Other sickle cell issues:

OTHER MEDICAL PROBLEMS (CIRCLE)

Asthma	Near-sighted (myopia)	G6PD deficiency
Seizures	Other:	

ALLERGIES (CIRCLE)

None	Food	Medication	Environmental

REGULAR DOCTORS (FILL IN OR ATTACH BUSINESS CARDS)

Name:	Name:	Name:
Address:	Address:	Address:
Telephone:	Telephone:	Telephone:
Fax:	Fax:	Fax:

MY TYPICAL HOME TREATMENTS FOR PAIN (YOU AND YOUR DOCTOR SHOULD CIRCLE WHAT HELPS):

Drink more fluids	Rest	Relax
Use a warm pack	Listen to music	Massage
Acetaminophen	Ibuprofen	Codeine
Hydrocodone	Naproxen	

RECOMMENDED HOSPITAL TREATMENTS (YOU AND YOUR DOCTOR SHOULD CIRCLE WHAT HELPS):

Rest	Use a warm pack	Incentive spirometry
Relax	Massage	IV fluids
Drink a lot of fluids	Morphine	Ketorolac
Laxative	Anti-itch medication	Anti-nausea medication

Hydromorphone every ___ hours, or patient-controlled analgesia

Get out of bed 2-3 times a day, starting day 2

WHAT HAPPENS IF I DO NOT HAVE MEDICAL RECORDS OR A HEALTH PASSPORT?

Without your medical records, you may get incorrect or delayed treatment, including:

* a duplicate test or injection
* a medicine that triggers an allergic reaction
* a transfusion that triggers a transfusion reaction
* a waste of time trying medication doses or treatments again that did not work for you in the first place
* a delay while the doctors or hospital ask you to remember your medical history and ask for a copy of medical records from the other doctors or hospital

SPORTS

People with sickle cell disease are likely to do better in sports that reward concentration and skill rather than endurance. Golf, martial arts, cycling, target shooting, archery, bowling, table tennis and fencing are all good choices. Swimming in a heated pool is also recommended because of its low impact on the hip joints. "Extreme" or endurance sports (long-distance competitive running, for example), which push the body to exhaustion and cause dehydration, are likely to cause problems. Sports that involve cold temperatures (skiing, sky diving) or low oxygen (mountain climbing) will probably trigger sickle cell pain.

If you are active, you'll need to pay particular attention to your hip, where avascular necrosis is extremely common in young adults with sickle cell. This can be accelerated by repetitive injury from high-impact sports. Pain in the hip or knee should be evaluated by an orthopedic doctor with sickle cell experience. If you have been diagnosed with avascular necrosis of the hip, you should not participate in sports that involve repetitive jumping (basketball, dance, and gymnastics, to name a few) that may cause further injury to the hip joint.

To avoid exhaustion, take frequent breaks when playing. During vigorous play, taking a break every fifteen to twenty minutes both to rest and to drink usually will allow you to continue your activities without developing lactic acidosis. Physical education teachers or coaches may need a note from the family or a doctor to explain this situation.

HOBBY AND CAREER CHOICES

Live every day to the fullest and prepare for a life into adulthood. Preparation should be made for work, marriage, hobbies and meaningful contributions to society. Education and skills are very important. People with sickle cell are lawyers, teachers, computer programmers, artists, moms, and dads.

Jobs that require heavy activity or working outdoors in bad weather are not good choices for people with sickle cell disease. Professional sports that involve endurance performance are not likely to be good choices either. Aim for indoor jobs, flexible schedules or white-collar jobs. You will probably need good grades and college or a professional education. Performing arts can be a good choice. Some famous musicians had sickle cell disease.

Teens and young adults with sickle cell in Chicago were asked: What jobs would you need to avoid because of sickle cell? What are your dream jobs?

JOBS TO AVOID	DREAM JOBS
Mail carrier	Early childhood teacher
Construction worker	Pediatric nurse or certified nursing assistant
Warehouse	Pediatrician
Road worker	Radiologist
Gym trainer	Therapist
Marine biologist	Lawyer
	Accountant
	Court reporter
	Model, fashion designer, actress
	Court stenographer

REAL-LIFE CAREERS OF PEOPLE WITH SICKLE CELL DISEASE

- Lawyer
- Physician
- Psychologist
- Minister
- Teacher
- Gospel singer
- Electrical engineer
- Business owner
- Vice president of a multinational computer software company
- Public health policy-maker at the Centers for Disease Control
- NASA engineer
- Clinical research nurse
- Daycare center owner
- Accountant
- Journalist
- Computer programmer
- Disc jockey
- Professor
- Health education policy-maker at the National Institutes of Health

Widely considered one of the most influential musicians of the 20th century, Miles Davis also had sickle cell disease. Sickle cell caused him a lot of pain and hip joint problems. It did not stop him from playing great music and sponsoring others to bring forth new types of music. He had to get hip replacements starting in 1976.

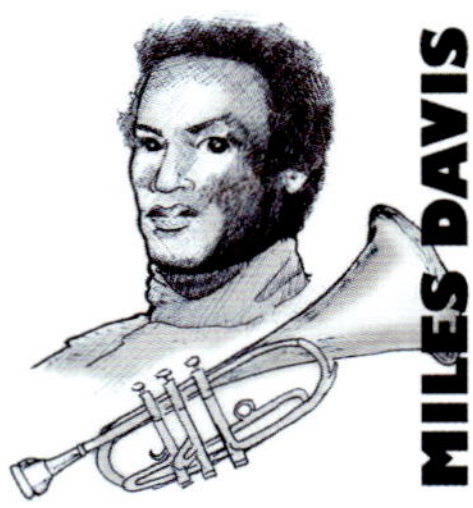

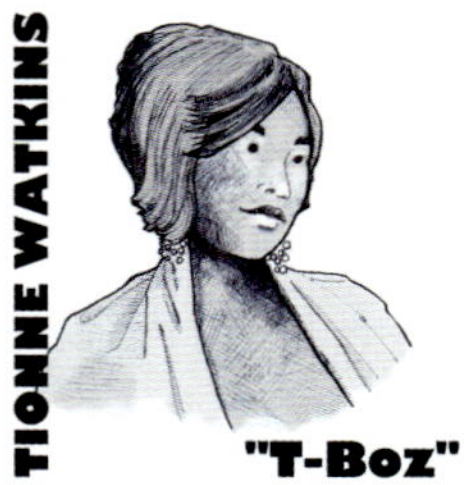

Despite hospitalizations at an early age due to sickle cell disease, Tionne "T-Boz" Watkins grew up to become a Grammy Award-winning musician as one-third of the successful R&B group TLC. She has also enjoyed a solo singing career, a reality-television show, has published a book of poetry and owned a children's clothing boutique.

AVOID INFECTION: FIVE TIPS TO HELP PREVENT INFECTIONS

Common illnesses, such as the flu, can quickly become dangerous for a person with sickle cell disease. The best defense is to take simple steps to help prevent infections.[1]

HAND WASHING

Washing your hands is one of the best ways to help prevent getting an infection. People with sickle cell disease, their family and other caretakers should wash their hands with soap and clean water many times each day. If you don't have soap and water, you can use gel hand cleaners with alcohol in them.

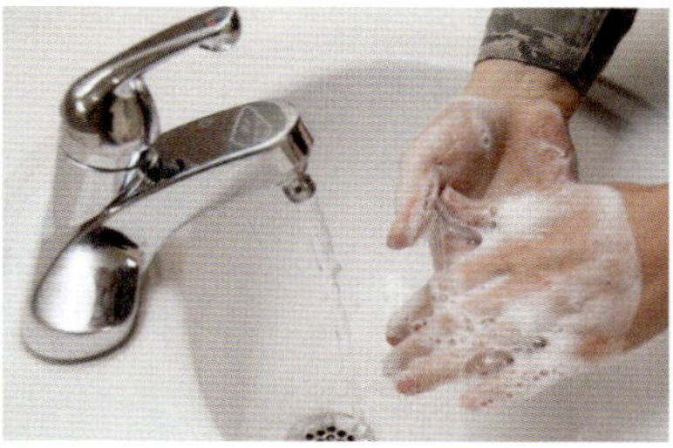

U.S. Air Force

Times to wash your hands:

BEFORE

* Making food
* Eating

AFTER

* Using the bathroom
* Blowing your nose, coughing, or sneezing
* Shaking hands
* Using public transportation such as buses and trains
* Touching people or things that can carry germs, such as:
    - Diapers or a child who has used the toilet
    - Food that is not cooked (raw meat, raw eggs, or unwashed vegetables)
    - Animals or animal waste
    - Trash
    - A sick person

---

1 *https://www.cdc.gov/ncbddd/sicklecell/healthyliving-prevent-infection.html*

FOOD SAFETY

Salmonella, a bacteria in some foods, can be especially harmful to children with sickle cell disease. How to stay safe when cooking and eating:

* Wash hands, cutting boards, counters, knives, and other utensils after they touch uncooked foods.
* Wash vegetables and fruit well before eating them.
* Cook meat until it is well done. The juices should run clear and there should be no pink inside.
* Do not eat raw or undercooked eggs. Raw eggs might be hiding in homemade hollandaise sauce, Caesar and other homemade salad dressings, tiramisu, homemade ice cream, homemade mayonnaise, cookie dough and frostings.
* Do not eat raw or unpasteurized milk or other dairy products. Make sure these foods have a label that says they are "pasteurized."

REPTILES

Salmonella can also be carried by reptiles. Make sure children stay away from turtles, snakes, and lizards.

VACCINES

Vaccines are a great way to prevent many serious infections. Children with sickle cell disease should get all the regular childhood vaccines, plus a few extra.

The extra ones are:

* Flu vaccine every year after six months of age.
* A pneumococcal vaccine (called 23-valent pneumococcal vaccine) at two and five years of age.
* Meningococcal vaccine (for some children).
* Conjugated pneumococcal vaccine PCV-13 (at least once).

Adults should have the flu vaccine every year, as well as the pneumococcal vaccine and any others recommended by a doctor.

PENICILLIN

Take penicillin (or another antibiotic prescribed by a doctor) every day until at least five years of age.

GET SUPPORT

Find a patient support group or community-based organization that can provide information, assistance and support.

HOW FRIENDS CAN HELP

Share your feelings with friends and family—tell your friends and family if you are feeling stressed. They might be able to help. It is important that a friend be aware of your condition. In the event of an emergency, people with sickle cell should have someone who is able to contact their family or a physician if they are unable to do so themselves.

SUMMER CAMP

Camp activities can help sickle cell children learn lifetime coping skills. Tell your camp counselors about common triggers for sickle cell pain:

* Dehydration
* Extremes of temperature, especially chilling the skin
* Exhaustion (acidosis)
* Infection
* Stress
* Weather changes

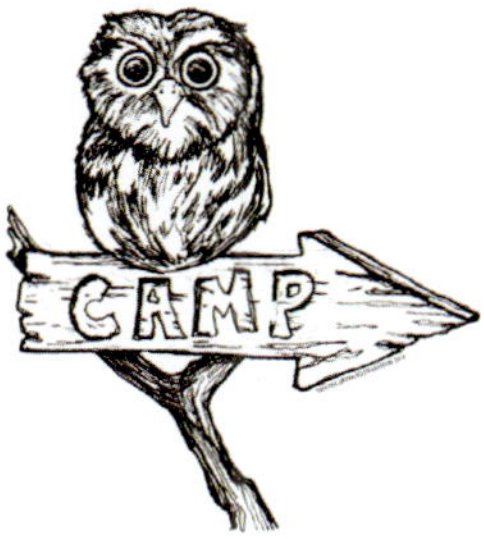

Camp counselors should keep the following in mind for campers with sickle cell:

* Be flexible with activity schedules. Allow the campers to take rest breaks and drink often.
* Carry fluids and encourage campers to drink often. In hot weather, seek shade and wear hats. Watch out for chilling during swimming—swimming in unheated pools is almost certain to trigger sickle cell pain in some children. Even in a heated pool, children with sickle cell

should take breaks after swimming about twenty minutes to dry off and warm up. Watch out for chills from excessive air conditioning—adjust temperature and/or allow campers to add layers of clothing.

* Help campers understand the consequences of overdoing it. Staying up late and/or playing too hard may lead to days of pain. Enforce rest breaks and reasonable bedtimes. Counselors with SCD should try to be role models for responsible behavior and not be afraid to ask for help or breaks. Plan staffing flexibility so that these counselors can call in a backup or substitute rather than suffering and "soldiering on" for the kids to the detriment of their own health.
* Help campers learn to sense their own body's warning signs. Try to head off pain or fatigue with rest, fluids and maybe pain medicine, and help the group to be supportive of fellow campers.
* Help campers remember to take their daily medications. Most will have to take a folate pill once a day. Some have to take penicillin, amoxicillin, or other antibiotics, twice a day, as regular prevention. Many have asthma medicines, which may be taken on schedule, plus as needed for activities. Some have iron chelation medicine. Desferal needs to be hooked up to a needle in the skin every night. Exjade is dissolved in liquid and taken as a drink. Jadenu can be a tablet or sprinkle granules. These iron chlelation medicines need to be stressed as an important treatment that should continue at camp.
* Enuresis—bed-wetting is very common due to effects of sickle cell on the kidney. Some camps put down absorbent disposable pads ("chucks") on the beds to avoid wet sheets. Some camps routinely change all the sheets on all the beds every day so there is no stigma for wet sheets. Some camps allow campers or counselors to do their own laundry inconspicuously.
* Group support and learning from peers are extremely valuable aspects of the camp experience. These are important reasons for children with sickle cell disease to go to camp together. As children gain experience with coping, they may be ready for camp with children with other chronic diseases or ordinary children.

AIR TRAVEL WITH SICKLE CELL DISEASE

Most people with sickle cell disease adapt well to air travel, but some can run into difficulties. Unfortunately, it is not always possible to predict if you will do just fine or be among those who have trouble flying. For this reason, it helps to know about potential problems so that you can take preventive measures or deal with them head-on if they should occur.

PRESSURIZED CABINS

Commercial jets fly at an altitude of around 30,000 feet, where the oxygen is extremely low, but their cabins are pressurized to keep the oxygen level equivalent to that at 8,000 feet. While this oxygen level is adequate for most children with sickle cell, you may need more. To play it safe, travel with major airlines and call ahead of time to find out what altitude the flight will reach and what procedures are in place for the use of supplemental oxygen. Keep in mind—even if you do experience complications from the low oxygen level, it does not mean you will have a problem with every flight.

DEHYDRATION

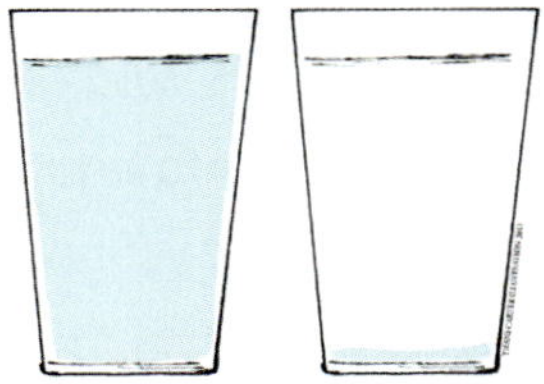

The air both in airports and on planes tends to be dry, so you will need to drink more than usual to avoid becoming dehydrated. This is easy enough to prevent—just pack an empty travel mug or sports bottle in your carry-on bag. After you pass through security, fill the mug or bottle with water for use in flight.

ALTITUDE AT DESTINATION

People with sickle cell probably will not experience trouble in cities with high altitudes such as Denver or Mexico City. The surrounding mountains are another story, though. Be aware that the higher you go, the more likely you are to develop pain or other sickle cell-related problems. You can take some control by going slowly and gradually to higher altitudes, by taking rest breaks and by drinking plenty of fluids.

MEDICAL CARE

Don't forget to take routine precautions, even if you are symptom-free. Be sure to take along documentation of your medical history in the event that you require emergency care—a record of past complications, treatments, allergies, and other medical problems is an invaluable resource for the doctors who treat you. Also have on hand the contact numbers for your primary healthcare provider in case you need to reach her. Another smart move—ask that same doctor if s/he can recommend a particular treatment center or provider at your destination where you can go in the event you need medical attention.

STRESS AND FATIGUE

Although indirectly related, stress and fatigue are often part of the travel experience. After arriving at a new destination, be sure to allow yourself time to rest and limit your activities as needed so that you do not become exhausted and trigger a pain episode. When traveling, build in a little flexibility and pack some fun things to do so that you can avoid boredom. Snacks can help, too. Do not forget books, art materials, music or videos.

IF I DO GET SICK, WHERE WOULD I GO FOR MEDICAL CARE?

It is a good idea to inquire before your trip, whether there are sickle cell centers in the vicinity of your destination. The National Alliance of Sickle Cell Centers maintains a list of centers on their website at *https://sicklecellcenters.org/member_centers*. Also check whether there are specific immunizations or preventive medications that you need to take (yellow fever vaccine? Meningitis vaccine? Anti-malaria medicine? Avoid drinking tap water?). A lot of travel health advice is available at *https://wwwnc.cdc.gov/travel*.

A group of sickle cell doctors in Paris, France, looked at their patients' experience with travel to Africa. They found that the biggest health risk is infection for sickle cell children traveling abroad. If there is malaria in the areas you will visit, make sure to take medicine to block malaria.

Adapted from drspock.com by Lewis Hsu, M.D., Ph.D. and Laura Jana, M.D., F.A.A.P. reviewed by Allan Platt, PA-C

MYTHS VS. FACTS

Myth: You can catch sickle cell disease from another person.

Fact: Sickle cell is not contagious. It is strictly an inherited disease, and only people who are born with this genetic anomaly can develop it.

Myth: Only African Americans get sickle cell disease.

Fact: Sickle cell affects many racial and ethnic backgrounds including African, Arabian, Israeli, Greek, Italian, Hispanic, Turkish, and Pakistani.

Although rare, there are blond-haired, blue-eyed children of Northern European extraction with sickle cell disease, and there is even a Chinese child in Hong Kong with sickle cell disease.

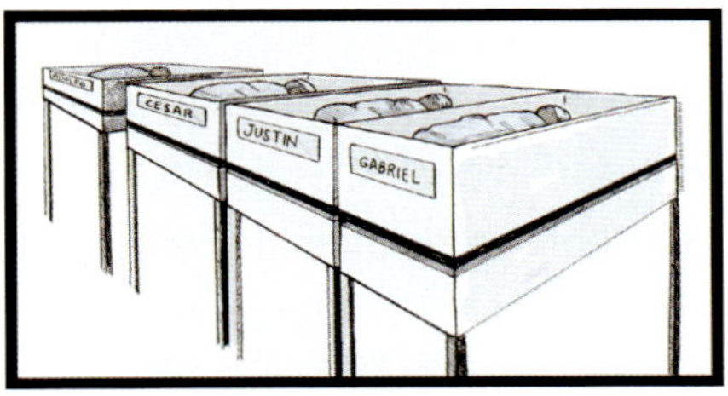

For this reason, in most American hospitals, all races now are screened at birth for the type of hemoglobin responsible for causing sickle cell disease.

Sickle cell disease suffers from a lot of misconceptions. Often thought of as an urban disease affecting only African-American children, in reality it is an international disease affecting many cultures around the globe and more than 30 million individuals worldwide. Here in the United States, 80,000 to 100,000 Americans suffer from sickle cell disease.

Sickle cell is the most common serious genetic disorder in the United States, more common than cystic fibrosis and hemophilia. But those diseases have high funding for research and many available medications while sickle cell disease does not. This means that we need to push for more funds, both from government grants and from donors.

Myth: If you have the disease, it means that you got the sickle cell gene from both parents.

Fact: This is true for one form of the disease (known as HbSS), but there are other types in which only one parent has passed on the sickle cell gene and the other has passed on a gene for another type of anemia, such as thalassemia, that combine to produce sickle cell disease. Other hemoglobin traits like hemoglobin C, hemoglobin D-Punjab, hemoglobin O-Arab can also combine to produce sickle cell disease.

Myth: I don't need to tell my doctors about having sickle cell trait, because this condition has no health implications at all.

Fact: Even though sickle cell trait does not cause problems as severe as sickle cell disease, there are still health concerns of which you should be aware.

Under extremely severe conditions—at the limits of human endurance, such as military desert-survival training or exercise at high altitude, or extremely harsh football practice in hot summer weather when still out of shape—people with the trait can develop severe health problems such as bleeding from the kidney and sickling in the spleen.

A blood test for diabetes (the hemoglobin A1C test) does not work correctly for people with sickle cell trait. More rare problems for people with sickle trait include bleeding from the kidneys and a type of kidney cancer called renal cell carcinoma.

Problems can generally be prevented for people with sickle trait by drinking plenty of fluids, getting into good physical condition gradually, getting adjusted to high altitude before attempting vigorous activity, and taking rest breaks when the weather is hot.

However, most of the millions of people with sickle trait show no health problems and never know that they have this trait. This includes many world-class athletes and members of the military. Some of the famous World War II fighter pilot group known as the Tuskegee Airmen had sickle trait, and they helped prove that sickle trait does not cause performance problems for combat pilots.

When your child grows up, if she and her spouse both have sickle cell trait, they should be aware that their children could be born with sickle cell disease.

Myth: People with sickle cell disease cannot get malaria.

Fact: People with sickle cell disease can indeed contract malaria and may either die or suffer through it and survive, just like anyone else. However, people with sickle cell trait tend to be more resistant to malaria—the trait doesn't completely protect a person from infection, but it makes death from malaria less likely.

This survival advantage is believed to explain the worldwide pattern of sickle cell in many peoples who frequently are exposed to malaria, such as those who live in sub-Saharan Africa, around the Mediterranean and on the Indian subcontinent.

Myth: Nothing has changed in sickle cell treatment. It is the same for my child as it was for my uncle who died at a young age of sickle cell thirty years ago.

Fact: Sickle cell treatment has improved greatly in recent years. People with sickle cell now have a life expectancy of at least into their mid-forties due to several recent advances in care. Preventing infections and treating fever get most of the credit for this improvement in survival. Early detection of sickle cell through newborn screenings also improves survival of lung and spleen problems. In addition, screening with transcranial Doppler ultrasound has greatly reduced strokes in children.

Myth: Nothing is available to treat sickle cell disease.

Fact: Sickle cell treatment now is greatly improved compared to even five years ago. Hydroxyurea and glutamine are effective medications for improving sickle cell. Read more about them in section 2 of this book. Monthly blood transfusions can prevent most of the problems of sickle cell. Iron overload can be treated with oral chelator. Bone marrow transplants now can cure some sickle cell children who have immunologic-matched siblings to serve as donors, and gene therapy is beginning to produce promising results.

Myth: Research doesn't matter to me.

Fact: More treatments are coming for sickle cell and need research studies to confirm their usefulness. New types of transplants are in ongoing clinical trials, and a recent clinical trial in Paris brought about the cure of a fifteen-year-old boy from advances in gene therapy. Medical and scientific advances are happening every day around the world. Making sure that you and your doctor keep up-to-date with sickle cell research will allow you to enjoy the benefits of future medical advances.

Myth: All of sickle cell care is medical in nature and administered by doctors and other healthcare workers. Nothing is under our control as a family.

Fact: Actually, there is quite a bit a family can do to care for a child with sickle cell. Strike a balance between completely denying the presence of the disease and living in a bubble. They can learn to recognize problems early on, when medical treatment often is more effective, and they can take precautions to ward off pain crises. Building up a support system of friends and family can make a big difference in how much a child's life is affected by sickle cell.

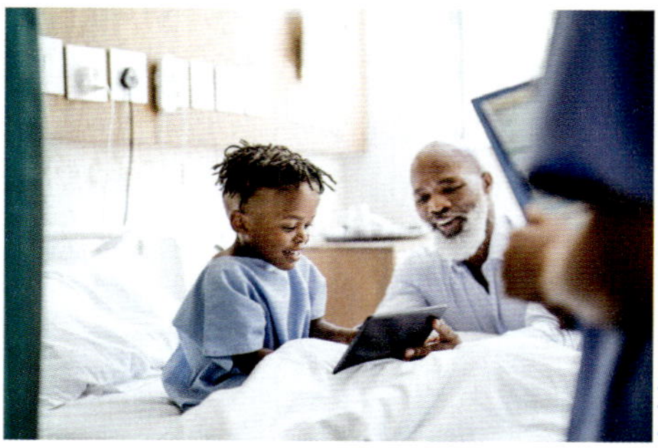

iStock / Getty Images

SICKLE CELL AROUND THE WORLD—NIGERIA

Nigeria is sometimes called "The Giant of Africa" because of its huge population (more than 160 million, the largest in Africa), vast land size, oil and other natural resources. It has one of the growing economies in the world, largely from oil in the Niger Delta in the southern part of the country.

Nigeria also has about 80,000 new babies with sickle cell disease SS every year, the highest rate in the world. Sickle cell centers focus on patient care, research and teaching in Lagos, Abuja, Ibadan, Kano, and other centers.

WHAT DOES IT MEAN TO INHERIT A SICKLE GENE?

Because this is a genetic condition, whether somebody gets sickle cell disease or sickle trait depends on what genes you get from your parents. Here is a little game to demonstrate what it means to inherit a sickle gene.

THE INHERITANCE GAME

You will need:

* Four small balls that are the same except that they are different colors
* For the instructions, we will pretend there are two blue balls and two white balls. If you do not have two colors of balls, you can use marbles or candies or pencils—any set of four things that come in two colors.
* Two bags that do not allow you to see what is inside. (A paper lunch bag can be used). Label or decorate one bag "Mother" and one bag "Father"

Pretend that different balls stand for different genes; one type of ball (blue) stands for normal hemoglobin genes and another ball (white) for sickle hemoglobin genes.

Every person has two genes for hemoglobin. A person with sickle trait has one normal hemoglobin gene and one sickle hemoglobin gene (one blue ball and one white ball).

If the mother has sickle trait, she has one normal and one sickle gene. Put one blue and one white ball in the bag labeled "Mother."

STORIES FROM KIDS LIKE YOU

Hi. I started at Boldrini Children's Hospital when I was only 2 months old. I've had a total of six surgeries. I am now not hospitalized because of pain but because of fever. I have already removed the spleen due to "sequestration" of the blood.

This why I am admitted to the hospital each time I have a fever.

I have also had my tonsils removed as well as my gall (bladder). I've had surgery on my foot because I was born with a club foot. I also have had surgery on the kidney and two others.

I just told you that I've not been hospitalized because of pain and also that normally I do not have much pain. However, when I do have a pain crisis, the pain is unbearable. It seems like I will not last.

Because of this illness, I have to take a drug called hydroxyurea. Besides having this disease I also have allergic rhinitis, asthma, sinusitis and bronchitis. I also take Benzetacil every 21 days.

When I was younger, I was hospitalized very often. It was about three times every three months. After I was 11 years old this decreased immensely. Last year I has only one hospitalization and I stayed only 3 days in the hospital. I hope to God that it diminishes more and more.

Formerly sickle cell anemia had no cure. I was very sad knowing that I was going to die with this disease. Hopefully in the future if I have this surgery I will no longer have this disease and I will be well.

Henrique, 14 years old

If the father has sickle trait also, he has one normal and one sickle gene. Put one blue and one white ball in the bag labeled "Father."

When the mother and father have a baby, the baby gets one gene from the mother and one gene from the father—reach into the bag and pull one ball from each and see what genes the baby has now.

What kind of hemoglobin condition do these genes give this baby? Choices are:

* Normal hemoglobin (two blue balls)
* Sickle trait (one blue ball and one white ball)
* Sickle cell disease (two white balls)

That's right! You learned how a mother and a father's genes can give a baby a new genetic combination. So you see that this is one possible combination from this imaginary mother & father who both have sickle trait. Another baby from the same parents could have any of the other combinations of genes, because with every pregnancy there is a random chance of each gene combination.

UNDERSTAND HOW SICKLE CELL DISEASE COULD AFFECT YOUR BODY

WHAT PARTS OF THE BODY ARE AFFECTED BY SICKLE CELL?

Since blood travels all through the body, sickle cell disease affects many different parts of the body. It can be scary reading about these problems, but try not to be nervous. Most people with sickle cell will not experience all of these complications. Also, if you know about these issues and you understand your body, you could prevent some of these problems or get help for them before they cause you too much trouble.

The following pages have information on how sickle cell disease affects different body parts and symptoms you should watch out for.

Adapted from www.childrensnational.org/sickle-cell

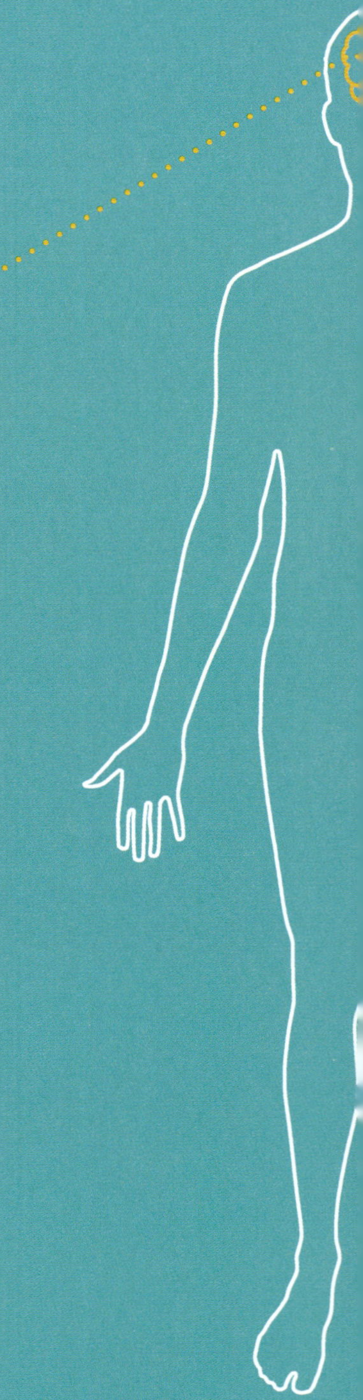

BRAIN

A stroke occurs when blood flow to the brain is blocked.

How do I know I might be having a stroke? What do I do?

Remember FAST to help check for signs of a stroke:

* **Face.** Smile. Does it look uneven or droop?
* **Arms.** Raise both arms. Does one side drift down?
* **Speech.** Repeat a simple sentence. Does it sound abnormal or slurred?
* **Time.** If you answer yes to any of the above questions then brain cells could be dying and you need urgent medical treatment.

Act fast. If you have signs of a stroke, immediately call 911 or emergency services.

People with sickle cell disease who have had a stroke are often started on regular schedule of blood transfusion to try to prevent them from having another stroke.

What is a TCD sickle stroke screening test?

Children with sickle cell disease can have a test called transcranial Doppler (TCD). This test measures the flow of blood to the brain and the risk of having a stroke. Children whose blood flows very fast when measured by TCD are more likely to have a stroke. Many of these children will get monthly blood transfusions to lower their risk of stroke.

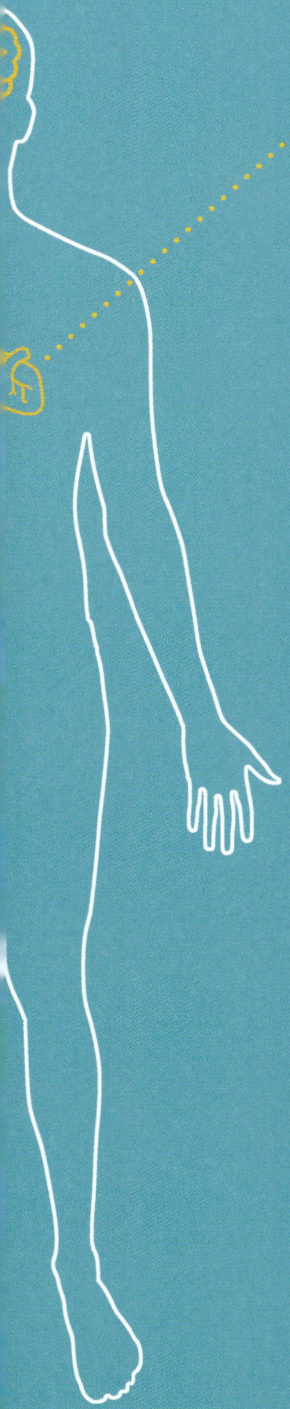

Brain by Grégory Montigny from the Noun Project
Heart by David Chapman from the Noun Project

HEART AND LUNGS

Pulmonary hypertension

Pulmonary hypertension is increased pressure in the blood vessels that go to the lung for oxygen transport. This increased pressure is caused by narrowing of these blood vessels.

To help understand pulmonary hypertension, think of two pipes with the same amount of water running through them.

Pipe #1 is big. Water easily travels through the pipe and does not push against it (low pressure).

Pipe #2 is small. Water has a more difficult time traveling faster through the pipe and pushes hard against it (high pressure).

Pulmonary hypertension is a problem because it can cause a strain on your heart. Symptoms of pulmonary hypertension include:

* New shortness of breath (dyspnea) with walking or climbing stairs
* Feeling tired all the time (chronic fatigue)
* Dizziness
* Fainting (syncope)
* Swollen ankles and legs (edema)
* Chest pain, especially during physical activity (angina)

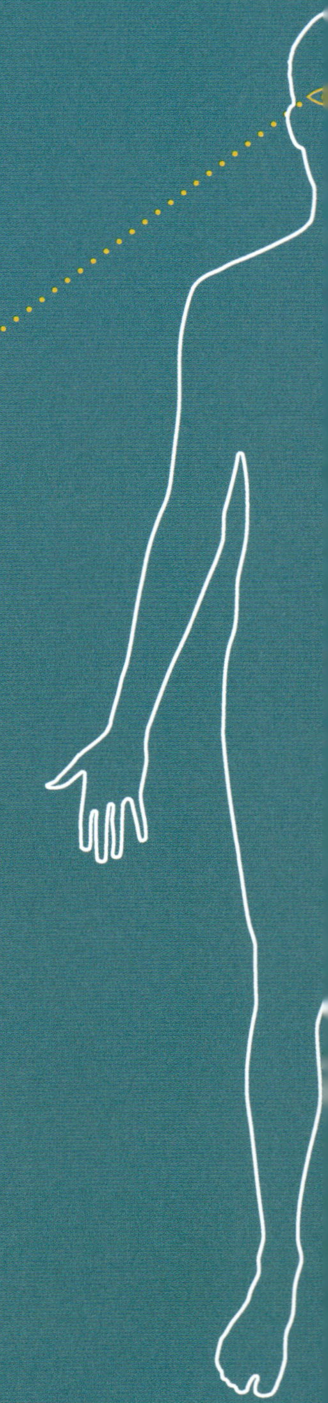

EYES

What is jaundice?

Jaundice means that parts of the body that are usually white have taken on a yellow color. The yellow color is most easily seen in the white part of the eyes (sclera).

The breakdown of red blood cells releases bilirubin, a yellow-orange substance. Faster breakdown of red blood cells means more bilirubin builds up. Many people with sickle cell always have some mild jaundice because their red bloods cells are broken down much more often than people who do not have sickle cell. This occurrence of jaundice is not concerning.

What if my eyes are more yellow than usual (increased jaundice)?

Your body might be destroying an increased number of red blood cells. Contact your doctor right away if you have increased jaundice plus urine that is dark brown, like the color of cola. Another explanation for increased jaundice is that you might be dehydrated. Drink more fluids, especially water. Finally, increased jaundice may indicate that your liver or gallbladder might have a problem. Jaundice that is due to liver or gallbladder problems is less common. However, if you have pain in your right side with the jaundice or increased jaundice that does not improve with rest and fluids, contact your doctor.

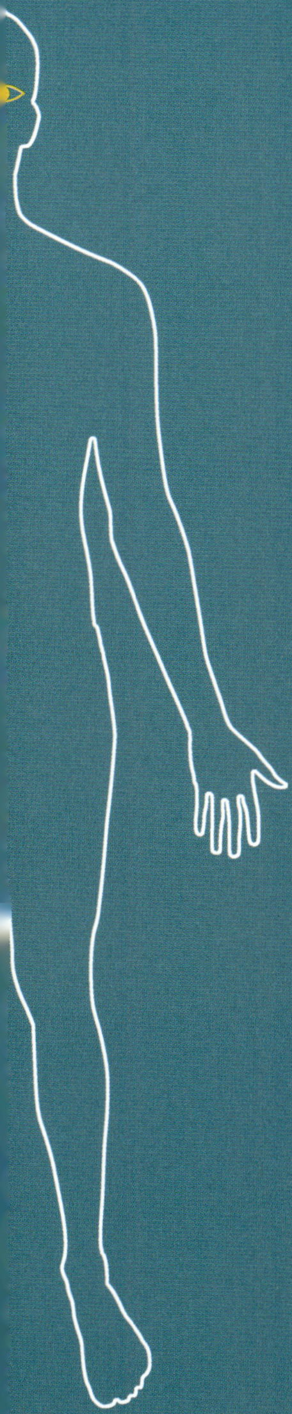

eyes by buheicon from the Noun Project

Retinopathy

Retinopathy means damage to the back of the eye, which controls your vision. People can develop different types of retinopathy for various reasons. Sickle cell disease can cause a specific type of retinopathy called sickle cell retinopathy. In the early stages of retinopathy, your vision might be perfect. However, retinopathy often gets worse, causing vision problems and even blindness. Fortunately, retinopathy can usually be treated by laser surgery before it causes vision problems.

People with sickle cell should see an ophthalmologist (an eye doctor) to look for retinopathy and treat it before it causes problems. It is very important to see the ophthalmologist every year starting at around age ten, even if you have 20/20 vision.

Sickle cell disease changes some of the blood vessel patterns in the retina. Normally, blood vessels branch out to supply the whole retina with blood flow. Blocked vessels can make a gap in the blood vessels that looks like a sunburst. Blood vessels become more twisted and curved, and some seem to disappear, like plucking out threads from a net. Extra blood vessels grow in to fill in the gaps, but sometimes the new vessels grow in bunched-up patterns that lift off the surface of the retina instead of simple networks on the retina. One of these bunched-up patterns is nicknamed "sea fan."

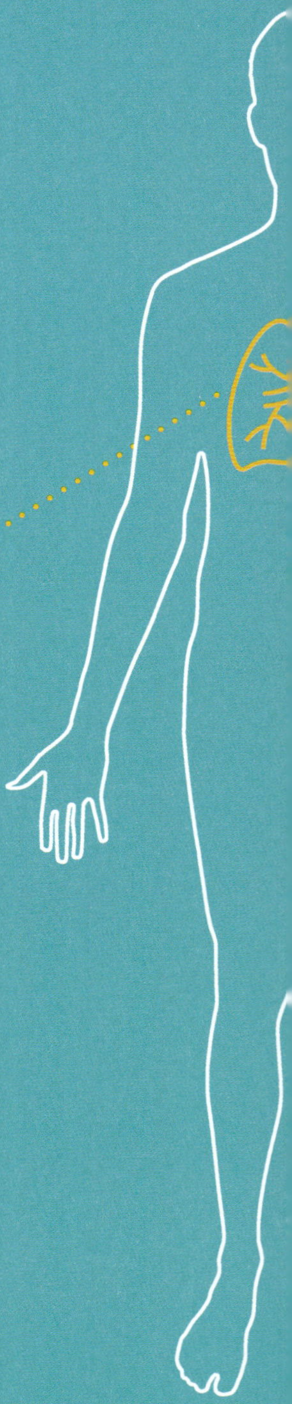

Acute chest syndrome

Acute chest syndrome (ACS) describes a type of sickle cell crisis involving the lungs. ACS is diagnosed by seeing a new infiltrate (evidence of a substance not normally present) on a chest X-ray. Some doctors may use the word pneumonia (inflammation of the lung) to describe this abnormality. In general, pneumonia in a person with sickle cell disease is the same thing as acute chest syndrome.

A person with acute chest syndrome has one or more of the following symptoms:

* Fever
* Cough
* Difficulty breathing
* Chest pain

It is very important to see a doctor if you have any of the above symptoms, because people with ACS can become very sick.

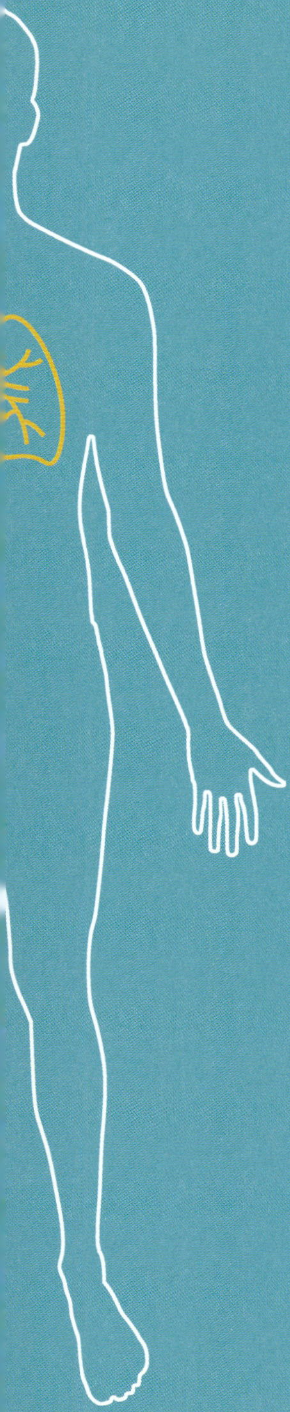

Lungs by karina from the Noun Project

How is acute chest syndrome treated?

Treating ACS involves helping to ensure that your body is still receiving enough oxygen. Supplemental (extra) oxygen is often given. Breathing treatment medications like the ones used for asthma may also be given to help improve lung function. Sometimes a blood transfusion is necessary to further help with oxygen transport. Since ACS may be triggered by an infection, treatment can also involve antibiotics.

How can I prevent acute chest syndrome?

One important thing that you can do to prevent acute chest syndrome is incentive spirometry. An incentive spirometer is a device that helps encourage you to breathe in deeply. By taking deep breaths, your lungs will better deliver oxygen and prevent vasoconstriction of the blood vessels going to the lung that can cause acute chest syndrome. If you are in the hospital for a pain crisis, you should try to use your incentive spirometer for ten breaths every hour while awake, or once every time you see a TV commercial, for example.

Another important thing you can do to prevent acute chest syndrome and other problems is to get your influenza (flu) vaccine every year. All people with sickle cell disease should get a flu vaccine before the start of the flu season in the early fall; flu vaccines are usually first available in September. You need to get the influenza vaccine every year because the influenza virus changes every year. The vaccine is specially made to protect against the most common strains of influenza virus of the current season.

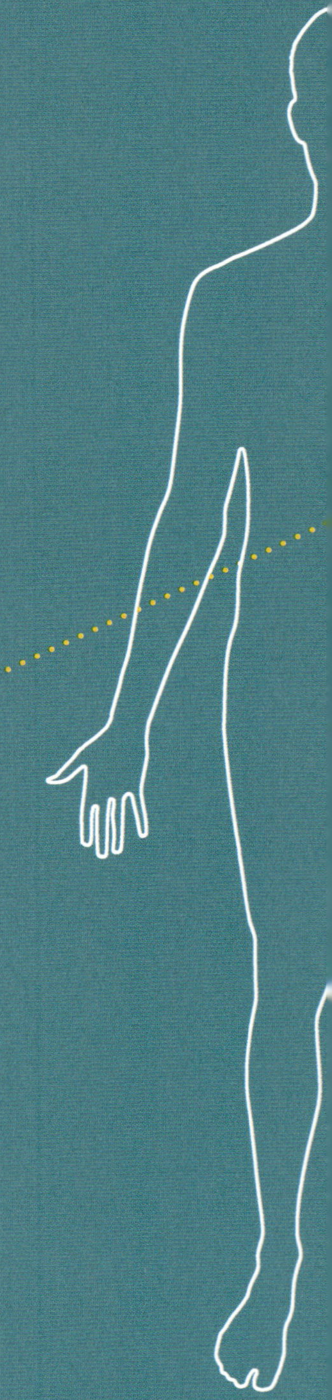

SPLEEN

The spleen is an organ in the left upper abdomen that removes old or damaged red blood cells. The spleen is also part of the immune system and helps fight certain infections.

Splenic sequestration is the sudden enlargement of the spleen due to trapping of red blood cells. This causes problems because fewer red blood cells are available to circulate in the rest of the body to transport oxygen. People with splenic sequestration need to be hospitalized and may need a blood transfusion.

After recovering from a splenic sequestration event, you may start chronic blood transfusion therapy or have the spleen removed (splenectomy) to prevent future episodes. Splenic sequestration usually only occurs in children with sickle cell disease before they develop functional asplenia.

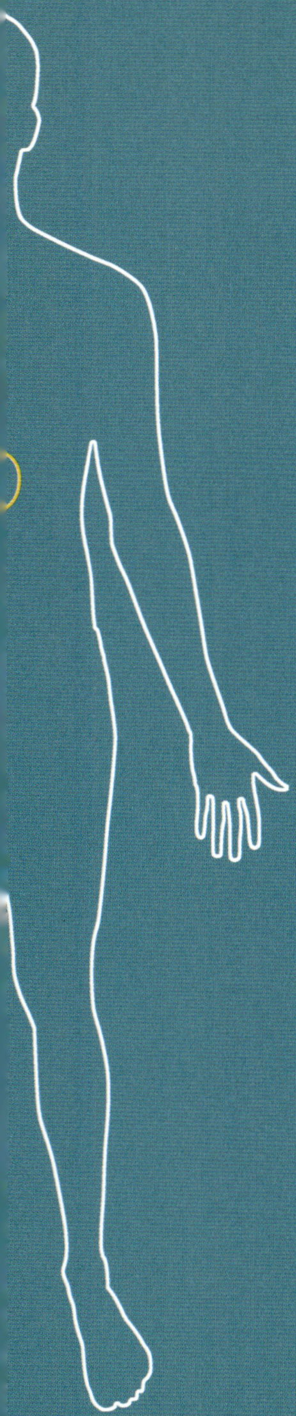

Spleen by IcoLabs from the Noun Project

Functional asplenia

The spleen in individuals with sickle cell disease usually becomes damaged over time by the many abnormal red blood cells traveling through it. Usually, by adolescence, the spleen in individuals with sickle cell disease stops working because of this damage. Functional asplenia simply means not having a working spleen.

No spleen—who cares?

People can live without a spleen. However, people who do not have a functioning spleen have an increased risk of certain infections, especially infections from bacteria called pneumococcus. Because of this increased risk, all people with sickle cell should see a doctor immediately if they have fever—an oral temperature above 101.3°F or 38.5°C. Fever could be the first sign of a serious bacterial infection that needs immediate antibiotic treatment, so go to the emergency room.

As a child you should have taken penicillin, an antibiotic to prevent blood infection by the bacteria called pneumococcus. It is recommended that all children with sickle cell disease younger than five years old take penicillin everyday. It is also recommended that older individuals continue taking penicillin if they have had a past pneumococcus blood infection or had a splenectomy, which is surgery to remove the spleen.

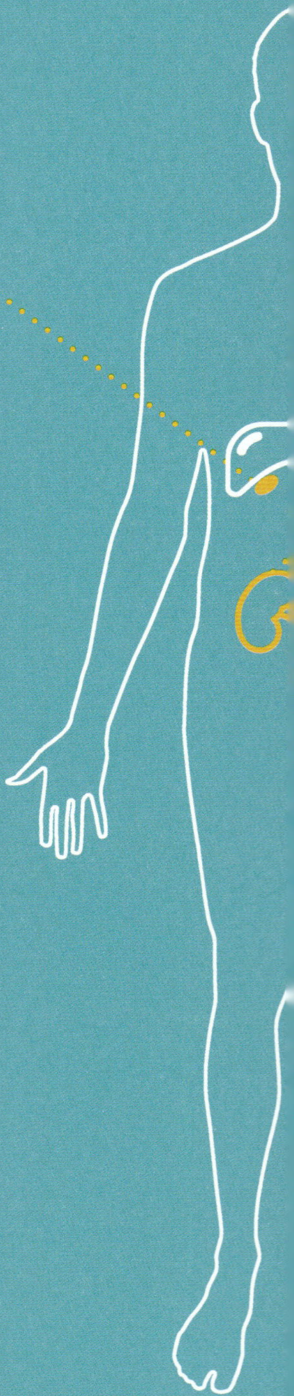

GALLBLADDER

The gallbladder is an organ in the right upper abdomen that stores bile, a fluid that helps with digestion.

Gallstones—people with sickle cell disease typically can develop types of gallstones called bilirubin gallstones. Bilirubin is a yellow substance made when hemoglobin in red blood cells is broken down. People with sickle cell disease have elevated bilirubin levels because of the constant break down of damaged red blood cells. This bilirubin can then collect to form gallstones. A few gallstones may not cause any problems, but over time, gallstones can block the flow of bile out of the gallbladder causing two problems:

Biliary colic—this is the word used to describe the abdominal pain caused by gallstones. People with biliary colic can have severe abdominal pain located in the right upper abdomen. Often this pain is worse after eating fatty meals, but then goes away.

Cholecystitis—an infection of the gallbladder that results from blocking the flow of bile. People with cholecystitis usually have a fever in addition to severe right upper abdomen pain and tenderness. People with cholecystitis need treatment in the hospital with antibiotics.

If you are having significant problems from gallstones, the treatment is surgical removal of the gallbladder (cholecystectomy).

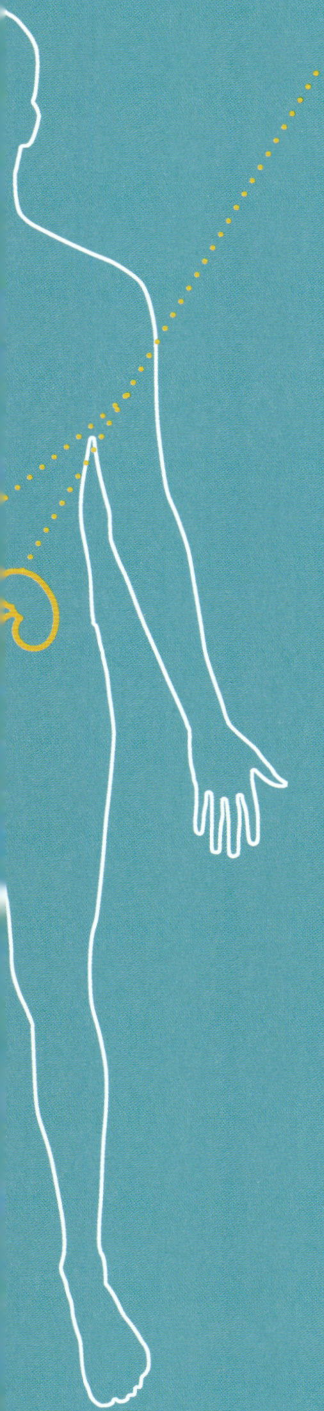

Liver by Andre Buand from the Noun Project
Kidneys by Vectors Market from the Noun Project

KIDNEYS

The kidneys filter blood, removing waste to create urine.

Sickle cell nephropathy

Sickle red blood cells can damage the kidney so that it is unable to filter your blood properly. This kidney damage is called sickle cell nephropathy. The first sign of this damage is protein in the urine (proteinuria). People with early sickle cell nephropathy have no symptoms, but they can later develop renal failure, which means that the kidneys no longer work. Renal failure can cause dangerous levels of different electrolytes in the blood since the blood is not properly filtered. People with renal failure must go on dialysis or have a kidney transplant.

What to do if you have proteinuria

If you have proteinuria, then you likely have early kidney damage. You should see a kidney specialist (nephrologist) to get started on medication to slow down this damage to the kidney.

Why is my urine so dark?

People with faster breakdown of red blood cells release more hemoglobin into the blood. If your body has time to process the hemoglobin to bilirubin, the bilirubin will show up in your urine as a yellow-orange color. If your body has less time to process the hemoglobin, it will become met-hemoglobin and your urine will be a dark brown color like cola. Finally, if your body has no time to process the released hemoglobin, your urine will be red.

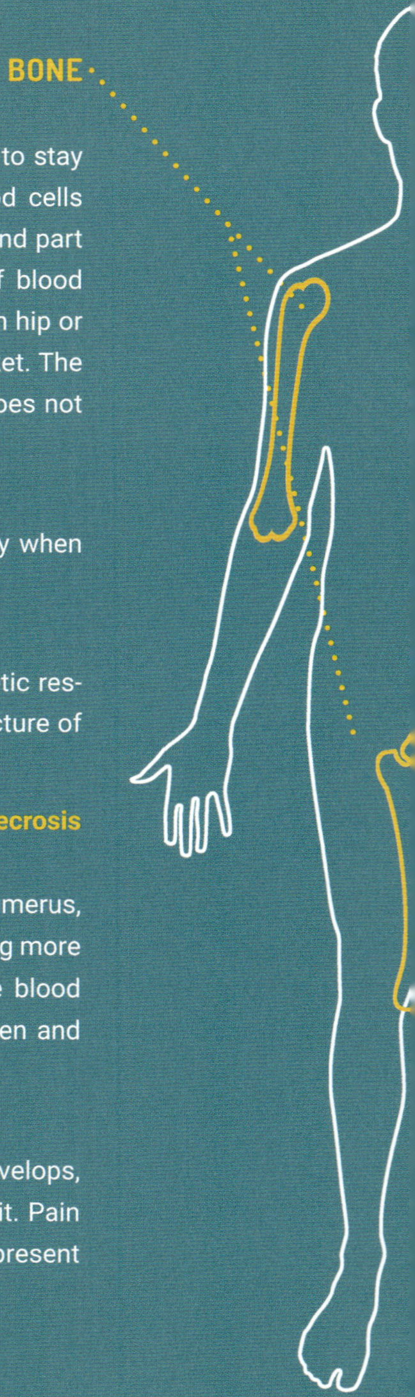

Avascular necrosis (AVN)

Bones, like other organs in the body, need blood to stay alive and healthy. Unfortunately, sickle red blood cells can sometimes block the blood supply to the round part of either the hip or shoulder bone. This lack of blood flow causes the bone to die, resulting in long-term hip or shoulder pain. The normal joint is a ball-and-socket. The damaged joint might have a flattened ball that does not fit well into the socket anymore.

How do I know whether I have AVN?

Sometimes early AVN causes hip pain, especially when you bring the knee toward your chest.

How is AVN diagnosed?

The best way to diagnose AVN is through magnetic resonance imaging (MRI). MRI takes a very good picture of the joint without any radiation.

What happens to the blood supply in avascular necrosis in sickle cell disease?

The ends of some bones, like the femur and humerus, have a pattern of blood vessels that makes sickling more likely. The sickle red blood cells slow down the blood flow. The bone tissue does not get enough oxygen and the bone tissue dies.

What are the symptoms?

Early AVN might have no symptoms. As AVN develops, the joint becomes painful when weight is put on it. Pain usually increases gradually with time and may be present even when resting.

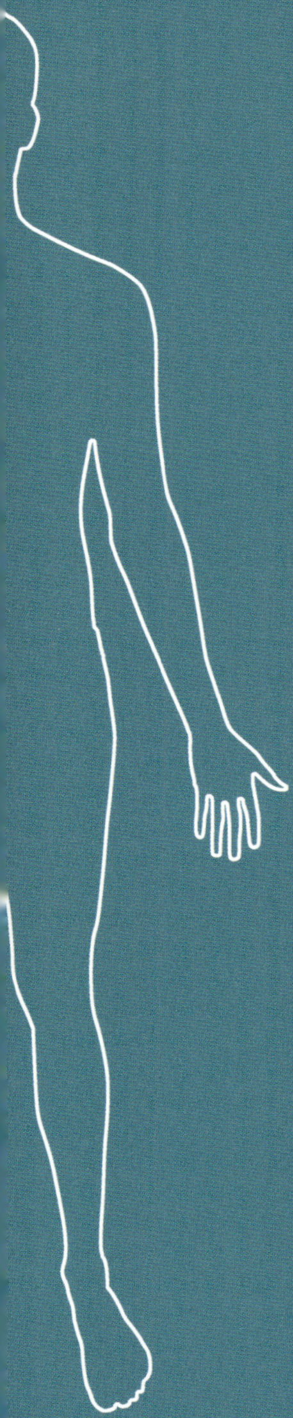

Bone by Philip Glenn from the Noun Project
femur by priyanka from the Noun Project

The pain that people feel with AVN is because of the bone-to-bone contact once the bone tissue is gone. Once it worsens, the loss of bone tissue can cause the bone joint to collapse. Eventually the joint may become very distorted and permanently painful. Eventually, joint function can be reduced. For example, your hip joint might not bend enough to sit normally, or your shoulder joint might not allow you to brush or comb your hair.

How is AVN diagnosed?

Early AVN does not show up on an X-ray. Your doctor would most likely recommend an MRI to see the damage. Later diagnoses can rely on X-ray.

Treatment options for AVN

The treatment for AVN differs depending on the case. Your doctor will most likely recommend some type of physical therapy such as:

* reducing weight on the hip joint—use crutches or change activities
* flexibility and strengthening exercises
* safe, moderate exercise
* heating pads to increase blood flow

For late AVN, surgery can replace the damaged bones with an artificial joint. For early AVN, other types of surgery are being studied to see whether the bone damage can be slowed.

Preventing AVN

* avoid joint impact—sports like trampoline are not a good idea
* keep your joints flexible
* reduce sickling by staying hydrated
* avoid obesity

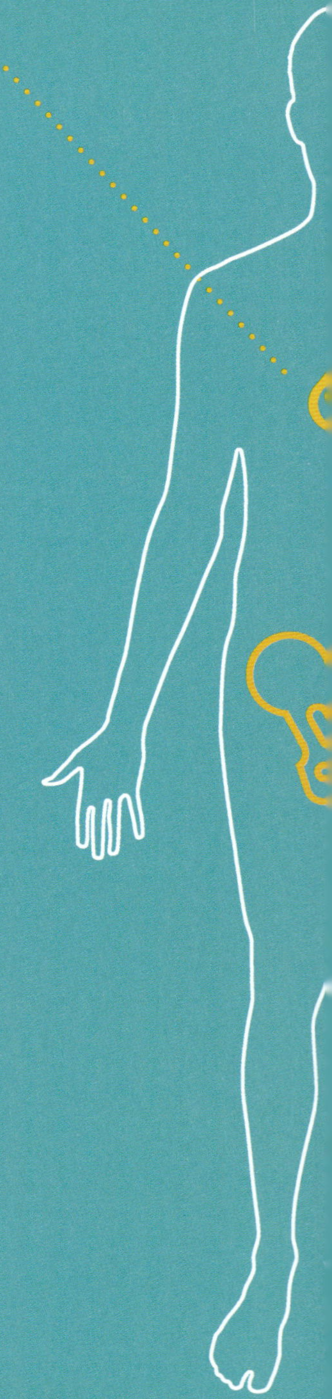

Blood transfusions can be life-saving for people with sickle cell disease in emergency situations such as severe acute chest syndrome. Chronic blood transfusions (scheduled transfusions every 3–4 weeks) are also important for individuals who have had a stroke. While blood transfusion therapy is very helpful, transfusions also have risks such as alloimmunization and iron overload.

Alloimmunization

The immune system is like a national army protecting your body from foreign invaders. Its function is to search for and destroy all things in your body that are not you, like bacteria and viruses. One weapon the immune system makes to attack pathogens is antibodies. Antibodies are like little missiles that attach to foreign particles and mark them as an enemy to be destroyed.

What does the immune system have to do with blood transfusions?

The immune system can sometimes identify lifesaving donor cells as foreign since your body did not make them. When this process happens, your body makes antibodies against the donor cells. For example, when an individual has made antibodies against a particular red blood cell, if he or she receives a blood transfusion of that type of red blood cell, it would be destroyed and could cause major problems. These antibodies make it more difficult to obtain a blood donor match.

Just like it is crucial for you to know your allergies to medications, it is very important to know if you have developed any antibodies to donor red blood cells. This information can help find the best blood for you in the blood bank next time you need a transfusion. Information about alloantibodies to red blood cells should be on a medical alert bracelet that can "speak for you" when you are in an emergency situation.

Iron overload

Iron is an important mineral used by your body. However, too much iron causes problems. Blood contains iron, so when you receive a blood transfusion, you also receive a significant amount of iron. Your body does not remove iron well, so over time if you have had many blood transfusions, the amount of iron in your body can rise to dangerous levels. In particular, iron can cause problems in the heart, liver, and endocrine glands.

How do you get rid of iron?

If your iron level reaches a certain level, you should start taking a medication called Exjade to remove iron. It is very important to take this medication every day to bring the iron in your body to a safe level.

BONE MARROW

Bone marrow is the "factory" that produces the different types of blood cells: white blood cells, red blood cells, and platelets.

Aplastic crisis

Aplastic crisis occurs when the bone marrow shuts down and stops making blood cells. Some viral infections can cause this aplastic crisis and temporarily stop the production of blood cells. People with sickle cell disease need to constantly make red blood cells since their red blood cells do not typically live as long. When the production of red blood cells stops, the number of red blood cells in the body can drop to a dangerously low level.

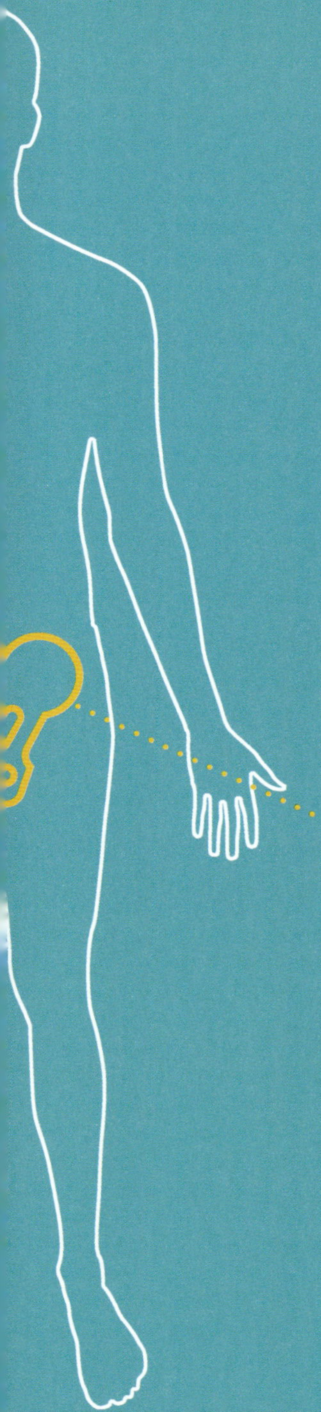

Pelvis by Tyler Hanns from the Noun Project

PRIAPISM

Priapism is an unwanted, prolonged erection of the penis. It can last for hours and often causes pain. Priapism does not occur because of sexual feelings or desires. Rather, it occurs when red blood cells sickle and change the chemistry of the blood, causing a blockage of normal blood flow draining from the penis. It can occur in all age groups. However, it usually affects males between the ages of 5 to 10 years and 20 to 50 years.

What causes priapism?

Priapism can occur in 42% of all males with sickle cell. It can also occur with other conditions (leukemia, cancer of the blood, malaria, injury, or certain medications). An erection that lasts over four hours can cause permanent damage to the penis. If untreated, priapism can cause impotence, which means that a man is unable to have an erection for sex.

What should I do if I have an erection that won't go down?

If you have a persistent erection, you should:

* Try to urinate.
* Drink plenty of fluids.
* Take pain medicine.
* Do some light exercise, such as walking.
* Put a cool towel on your penis.

If you have an erection that lasts longer than half an hour, then you need to immediately go to the emergency room, where you should receive IV fluids and pain medicine. If the erection remains, then a urologist (a surgeon who specializes in the penis) may need to give you an injection.

It is very important to go to the hospital if you have priapism. Do not ignore it or try to just deal with it at home. If you have priapism and wait more than two hours to go to the ER, you could cause irreversible and severe damage

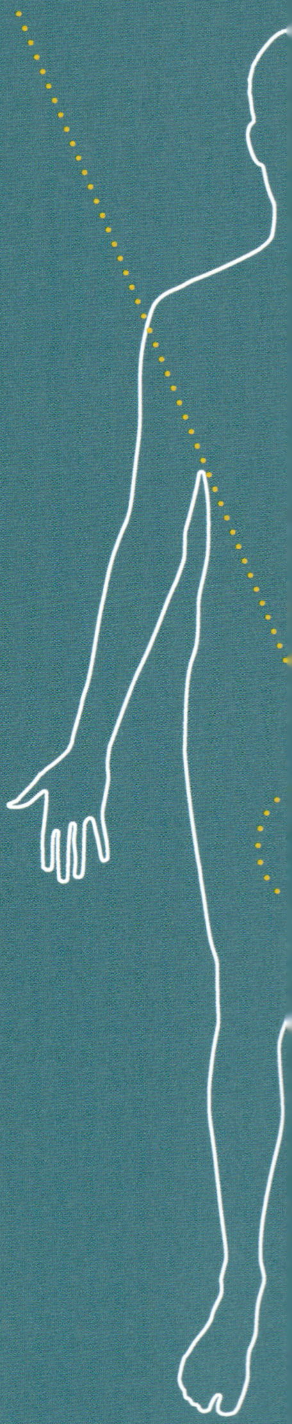

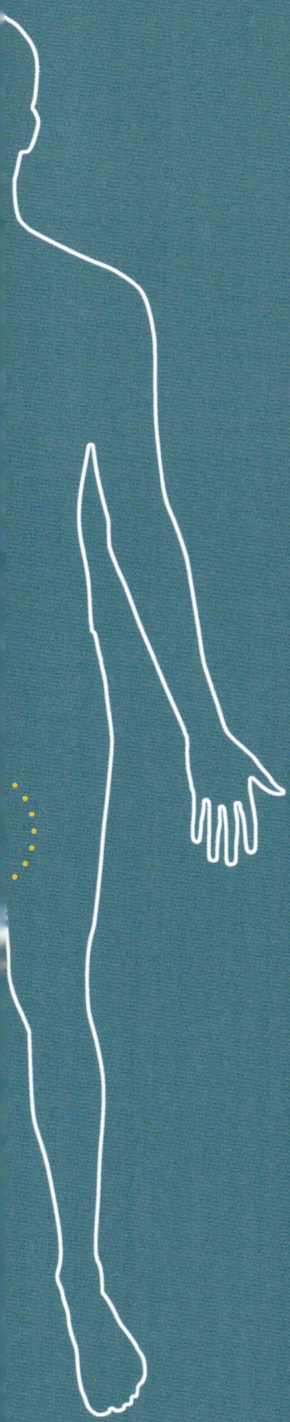

to your penis and maybe erectile dysfunction. Priapism is serious and not your fault; do not feel embarrassed to get help for it.

How is priapism treated?

If you receive treatment within four to six hours, the erection can almost always be reduced with medication. If the erection has lasted less than four hours, decongestant medications, which may decrease blood flow to the penis, may be very helpful. Other treatment options include:

Intracavernous injection: During this treatment, drugs called alpha-agonists are injected into the penis, causing the veins to narrow, reducing blood flow to the penis and causing the swelling to subside.

Aspiration: After numbing the penis, doctors will insert a needle and drain blood from the penis to reduce pressure and swelling.

Surgical shunt: A shunt is a passageway that is surgically inserted into the penis to divert the blood flow and allow circulation to return to normal.

If you suspect that you are experiencing priapism, you should not attempt to treat it yourself. Instead seek emergency help as soon as possible.

Is it safe for me to masturbate?

Masturbation is safe and usually does not cause priapism. If you have any concerns about having sex or masturbating, talk to your doctor.

Will I be able to father children?

Men with sickle cell disease are more likely to have problems with fertility and may have a more difficult time getting a woman pregnant, because sickle cell disease can affect sperm. However, men with sickle cell can get a woman pregnant and father children. If you have concerns about your ability to father a child, talk to your doctor.

PREGNANCY

Can women with sickle cell disease have a healthy pregnancy?

Yes, with early prenatal care and careful monitoring throughout the pregnancy, a woman with SCD can have a healthy pregnancy. However, women with SCD are more likely to have problems during pregnancy that can affect their health and that of their unborn baby. Therefore, they should be seen often by their obstetrician, hematologist, or primary care provider. You may also need to seek a special service called the "high-risk OB team."

During pregnancy, SCD can become more severe and pain episodes can occur more frequently.

A pregnant woman with SCD is at a higher risk of preterm labor and of having a low birth weight baby.

What should someone with sickle cell trait or sickle cell disease do if he or she is planning to have a baby?

A woman and her partner should get tested for sickle cell trait if they are planning to have a baby. Testing is available at most hospitals or medical centers, from SCD community-based organizations, or at local health departments. If a woman or her partner has sickle cell trait, a genetic counselor can provide additional information and further discuss the risks to their children.

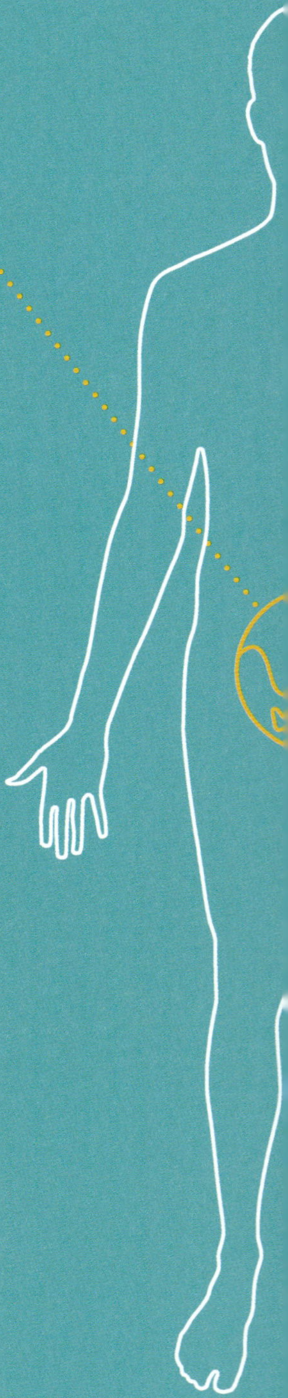

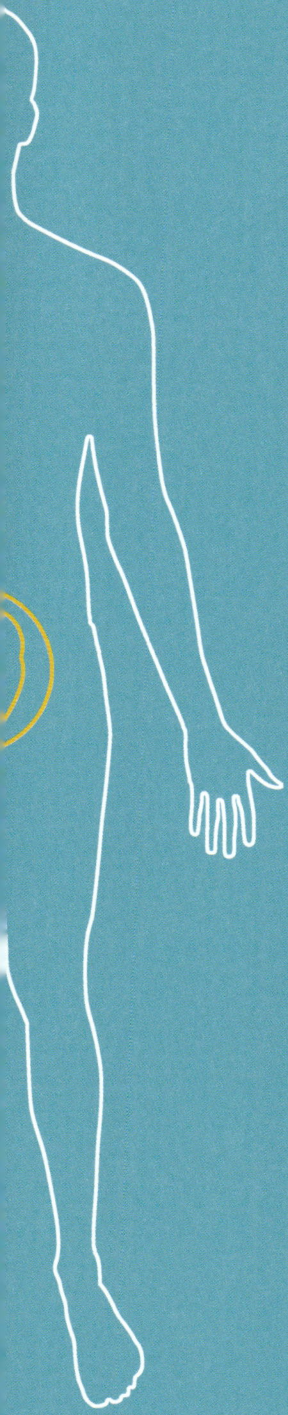

embryo by Laymik from the Noun Project

A woman or man with sickle cell disease should not have a baby while on hydroxyurea. This anti-sickling medicine causes birth defects in lab animals. Hydroxyurea has not caused birth defects in people with sickle cell, in nearly twenty pregnancies reported so far, but there were some spontaneous miscarriages.

Will someone with sickle cell trait or sickle cell disease have a baby with sickle cell disease or sickle cell trait?

During pregnancy, prenatal testing can be done to find out if a baby will have SCD, sickle cell trait, or neither one. The prenatal tests called chorionic villus sampling (CVS) and amniocentesis often are used to find out if the baby will have the disease or carry the trait. These tests usually are conducted after the second month of pregnancy.

(http://www.cdc.gov/ncbddd/sicklecell/documents/SCD%20factsheet_SCD%20%20Pregnancy.pdf)

MENSTRUAL PERIODS, CRAMPS, AND BIRTH CONTROL

Menstrual periods and bleeding may not always be regular for any teenage girl. Often obstetricians and gynecologists—doctors who specialize in the female reproductive system—will tell their patients to expect one to two irregular periods per year – that this is fairly normal. However, if a pattern develops with consistent heavy bleeding (having to change your pad or tampon more than six times per day), you should tell your doctors. Heavy bleeding can lead to anemia, a condition in which your body doesn't have enough red blood cells to carry oxygen to your organs and tissues. Symptoms include tiredness, dizziness, headache, and shortness of breath. If you have heavy bleeding, it's a good idea to always have extra pads or tampons and a change of underwear on hand. Having extra snacks and water available can help you avoid dizzy or faint spells.

Menstrual cramps are another common issue that many teenage girls deal with during menstrual periods. Cramps that are not related to sickle cell pain may occur from time to time; ibuprofen or naproxen can help, and applying heat to your lower abdomen with a heating pad or hot water bottle can also provide some relief. Regular exercise is another option that may help relieve menstrual cramps.

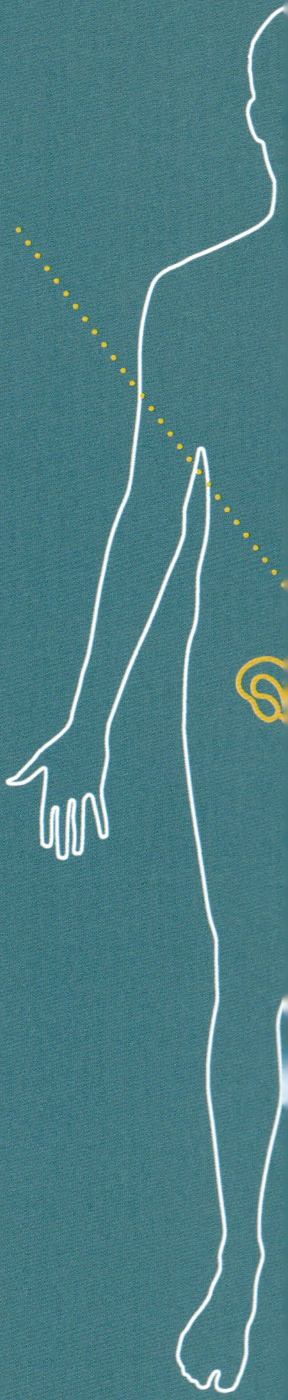

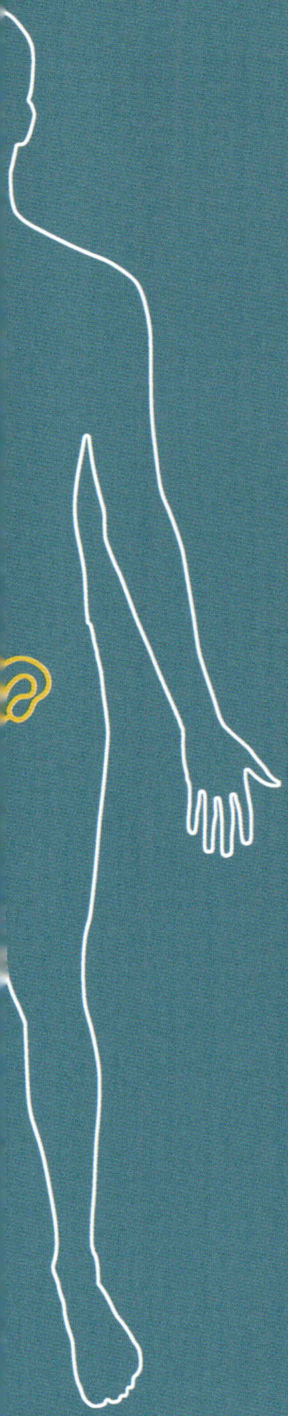

Uterus by ST from the Noun Project

If a pattern develops with sickle cell pain triggered by menstrual periods and cramping, doctors can give hormonal treatments to regulate your periods and avoid pain.

Hormonal birth control containing progestin, such as DepoProvera and Nexplanon, is generally chosen over estrogen-containing birth control pills for women with sickle cell disease since estrogen can increase the risk of developing blood clots. Hormonal IUDs (intrauterine devices) are also now being used with teen girls. The choice to use any medication is a personal one, and one you should talk about with your doctor and family. Birth control medication is discussed here in its connection and relevance to sickle cell disease.

Menstrual periods can be difficult enough for any teenage girl, let alone one with sickle cell disease. Make sure to take care of yourself when you're on your period by getting plenty of rest, drinking lots of water, and taking the pain medications your doctor recommends for you when you have cramps. You should also be aware that changes in your hormones before and during your period can cause feelings of sadness, depression, or anger, which is completely normal. Having these feelings on top of dealing with your sickle cell disease can certainly be overwhelming, so make sure to talk to your parents and your doctor if you are having a difficult time coping. They are there to help you through it.

STORIES FROM KIDS LIKE YOU

I do not remember when my parents found out about my sickle cell anemia. Also, I have no idea when I started taking Hydrea. But one thing has always remained clear in my memory: the hospitalizations, especially those that took me to the ICU and almost killed me.

My parents always supported me and, thanks to that, I was able to live much of my childhood normally with my physical limitations. I related to and enjoyed other people and made many friends. I was able to keep up my routine appointments just like an normal person. However, this only lasted until I was eight and I went to the ICU for the first time.

I vaguely remember why I was there. According to my parents, I was already in a coma when they took me to the hospital. However, I clearly remember the moment I woke up. The first thing I saw was a tube that went down my throat and hindered my breathing. Then I saw a number of devices which were connected to my body.

I immediately panicked and tried to get them out, but my body was too weak to react. The despair would have lasted longer if my mother had not been sleeping near my bed and held my hand.

Following this event the recovery was easy. I had the support of many friends, family and the nurses who cared for me. But that episode brought something into my life that no one could fix or forget: at only eight years old I discovered death. Over time this changed my way of living.

I managed to keep this decision of suffering along with its consequences until I reached adolescence. At that time I started to fail both physically and mentally. The crisis of pain intensified and the barriers that I had put in my mind when I was eight years old began to falter. Slowly the anguish began to leak out.

For a long time, while my body was suffering with pain crisis my mind resisted. That helped to facilitate the process of recovery and the hospitalizations.

However, in recent years it has become more difficult and even impossible flawed. My mind began to tire of fighting and the morphine which was applied in larger doses began easily devastating my mind and self control.

My way of dealing with death now turned into a poison that started leaking through the barrier that now was breaking. My parents and friends didn't know this side of me and consequently I felt very lonely. Every day I found it difficult to find reasons or forces to keep fighting and move on.

It has been less than a year since I had my last visit to the ICU. At this time the pain crisis followed by hospitalizations in important periods of my life like doing homework or taking tests have already shaken my hopes of graduating and of having a normal future.

Before I knew I was to go into the ICU I would spend the worst 24 hours of my life at home. I could not sleep. Instead, I would stay up in a kind of trance, feeling my body increasingly weaker and my life slowly ending.

Later I found out that I had had an acute chest syndrome but somehow had survived...but barely.

As soon as I woke up I found myself inside of a body weakened by disease and a mind completely destroyed by drugs. I looked like a cadaver and continued that way for a long period of recovery in which suicide and alcoholism were almost always present in my thoughts.

Now, I've recovered from this hospitalization. I am still trying to recover from the damage caused by my stubbornness. I am starting to trust people and I talk more about my experiences to other patients, and unlike what I imagined, these changes have made me well. I have begun to see sickle cell anemia in another way. I have found help and support in my friends and family, and finally I have begun to see reasons to fight against the disease and to believe in the existence of a future which overcomes the pain and the hospitalizations which have marked my life.

Ivo, 18 years old

UNDERSTANDING YOUR COMPLETE BLOOD COUNT (CBC) LAB RESULTS

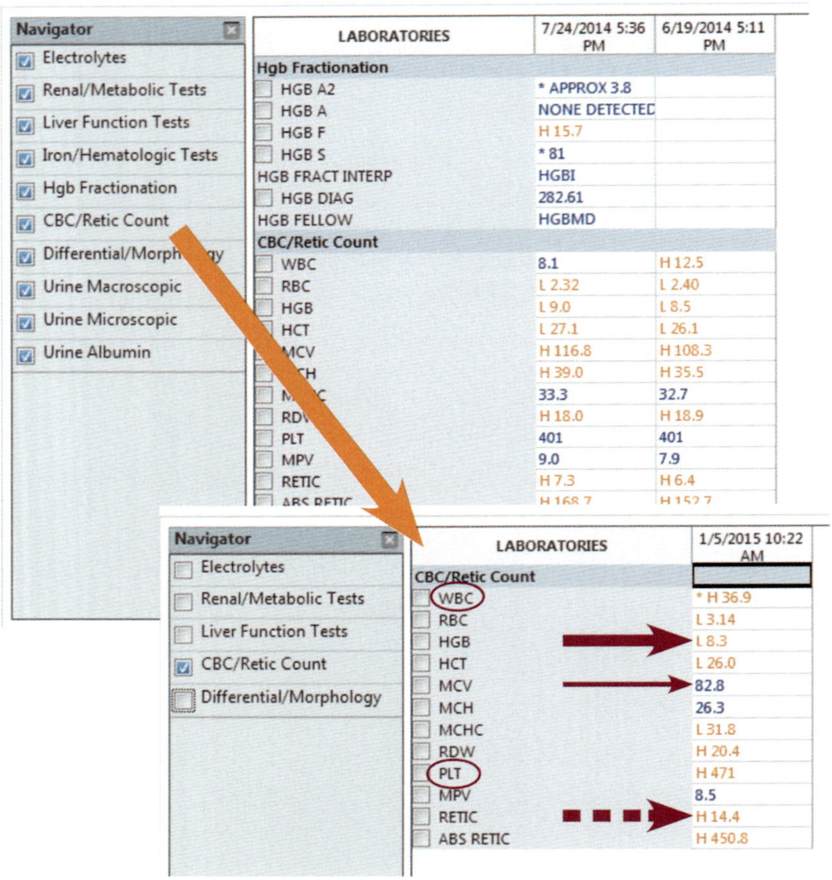

WHAT ARE THE KEY PARTS OF THE BLOOD COUNTS (CBC AND RETICULOCYTE COUNT) THAT I NEED TO UNDERSTAND WHEN REVIEWING MY LAB RESULTS?

The thickest arrow is on hemoglobin (Hgb or Hb). Lower numbers mean more severe anemia.

* The dotted arrow shows the reticulocyte percentage. Higher numbers mean more red blood cells are newly produced.
* The thin arrow is on Mean Cell Volume (MCV). Higher numbers mean

bigger red blood cells. Higher MCV is one of the helpful effects of hydroxyurea treatment.

* WBC is white blood cell count. Higher numbers mean inflammation or infection, or other stress to the body.
* Plt is platelet count. The platelet count can change in many sickle cell conditions.

THE LAB SHEET LISTS SO MANY RESULTS AS ABNORMAL. HOW DO I INTERPRET MY OWN CBC AND RETICULOCYTE RESULTS?

Having sickle cell disease makes many of your CBC results fall outside the ranges for people without any blood disorder. But looking over your CBC and reticulocyte results with your doctor can show you that many results always are the same when you are doing well. These are your own "base-line" CBC results.

DO THE CBC AND RETICULOCYTE RESULTS MEASURE PAIN?

It is important to know that pain cannot be measured with the CBC, the reticulocyte count, or with any other blood test available (as of 2019). You can still have sickle cell pain or other medical problems while your CBC and reticulocyte counts are "normal" for you, meaning they are at your baseline.

WHAT IF THE CBC AND RETICULOCYTE RESULTS ARE NOT AT MY BASELINE?

Interpreting why CBC or reticulocyte results are not at baseline in people with sickle cell can be very complicated. Not every doctor learns these skills. That is one of the biggest reasons why you should see a hematologist, or another doctor with a lot of experience treating sickle cell disease. Your hematologist can advise you on what to do and what treatment options are available to get your CBC and reticulocyte results back to your baseline.

STORIES FROM KIDS LIKE YOU

My name is Gabrielli and I have sickle cell disease. When I discovered that I had this disease I was two years old.

Well, I am going to tell you that it is something horrible to have, but if you take care of yourself correctly, take the medicines, don't get out in the cold and do all the things you know to do, like take the treatments on time, you won't have much pain. I have been here at the Boldrini Center for sixteen years.

When I was small I could not do the things that normal children do... (that is to say a normal child without any kind of sickness).

I could not play hide and seek because my heart has an opening between the valves (heart murmur) and I get very tired. In the hot weather my mother would not let me play in the swimming pool... She was afraid this would cause me pain. When the weather was cool I could not go out to play in my friend's homes.

Today I am eighteen years old. If one day I wish to marry I must bring my boyfriend here to Boldrini to do an exam to see if he has even a small chance of carrying this disease. If he does have any traces of the disease, and if one day we should want a baby, we cannot because the baby would be born with the disease. If he doesn't have any traces of the disease then we could have a baby.

However, I only want to have a child only after six months that I have stopped taking the medicine. Only then would I think about having a child. Even so I will take great care so I won't have pain while I am pregnant.

I believe a person who has sickle cell disease must take good care of himself and not stop taking the medicine. I stopped once and I know how I suffered later.

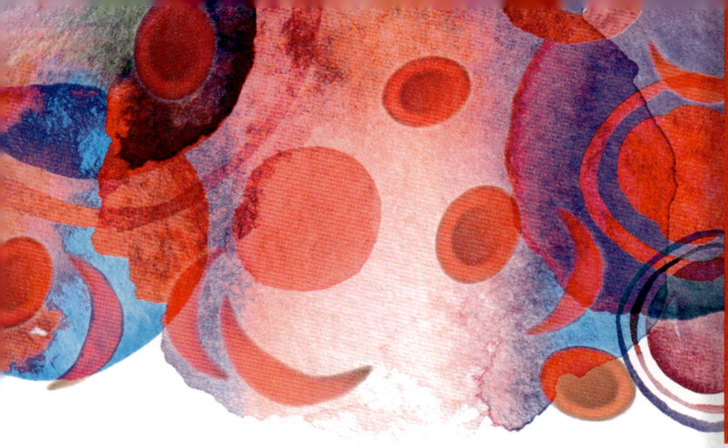

> Live your life without fear, but be diligent about your health.
>
> —Lisa, parent

SECTION 4

SICKLE CELL Trait

WHAT IS SICKLE CELL TRAIT?

If you have sickle cell trait, it means that of the two genes you inherited from your parents, one is for sickle hemoglobin and one is for normal hemoglobin. Normal hemoglobin is called hemoglobin A, and sickle hemoglobin is called hemoglobin S. Sickle cell trait is detected when a blood test called hemoglobin electrophoresis shows the presence of both hemoglobin A and hemoglobin S. Sickle trait is also called a "sickle gene carrier state" or "heterozygous for the sickle gene." **Sickle trait will NOT become sickle cell disease.**

SICKLE TRAIT USUALLY IS SILENT

The great majority of people with sickle trait never know that they have it. The most important thing is that they can pass along the sickle hemoglobin gene to their children. It is important that you know the hemoglobin genes of your partner. If you have sickle trait, you may have children with sickle cell disease if your partner also has sickle, thalassemia, or hemoglobin C trait.

COMMON MEDICAL PROBLEMS CAN BE AFFECTED BY SICKLE TRAIT

Certain types of the hemoglobin A1C test, which monitors diabetes, will give incorrect results in people with sickle trait, so other types of diabetes testing should be used instead. If you have sickle trait, there are slightly increased risks of urinary bladder infection and abnormal clotting (thrombosis).

SICKLE TRAIT WILL NOT BECOME SICKLE CELL DISEASE.

RARE MEDICAL PROBLEMS WITH SICKLE TRAIT

Under extreme conditions, the sickle trait red blood cells can actually sickle. Bleeding from the kidney is uncommon, but it can be caused by damage in the deepest parts of the kidney from sickle trait red blood cells. In very rare cases, bloody urine can be caused by a rare kidney cancer called renal medullary carcinoma, so bloody urine should be evaluated by a doctor.

If an eye injury causes bleeding in the eye, sickle trait blood cells can become trapped in the eye in a condition called hyphema. This blood can quickly cause vision loss if it is not flushed out. An eye specialist should be notified immediately about sickle trait and serious eye injury. The treatment can include close monitoring of the bleeding eye and eye pressure for several days.

Extreme exercise, at the limits of human endurance, can cause severe organ damage, sickling in the spleen, and sudden death. Heat, dehydration, altitude and asthma can increase the risk for sickling. The United States military found that this problem can be prevented by good hydration and proper coaching for progressive physical conditioning.

The super-strenuous activities that can cause problems for people with sickle cell trait include pushing yourself to the limits of human endurance (survival treks in the desert) or doing things foolishly, such as trying to exercise at high altitude (climbing in the Rocky Mountains) when dehydrated and out of shape, or suddenly beginning rigorous exercise (military basic training, summer training practice for American football teams) without being in shape. However, people who gradually get into good physical condition and pay attention to drinking plenty of fluids have been successful competitors at elite professional and Olympic sports.

A blood or DNA test can determine if you carry sickle trait. Meeting with a genetic counselor can help you understand what having sickle trait means and ease your worries about the stigma this might carry. It might help for you to know that sickle trait is more common than sickle cell disease and is prevalent in populations from many ethnic backgrounds, not just people of African descent.

SICKLE TRAIT HELPS PEOPLE SURVIVE MALARIA

DR. TONY ALLISON'S BLOOD SAMPLING SAFARIS ACROSS EAST AFRICA

Dr. Anthony C. "Tony" Allison was born in East Africa near the Great Rift Valley, where his father had migrated from Britain. As Allison was growing up, he saw that many people in East Africa had malaria, many people had anemia, and some had sickle cell disease. He also caught malaria himself. Tony loved to travel and learn about the geography of Africa.

Allison went to school in England to become a doctor, and he also earned a degree in biochemistry and genetics at Oxford University shortly after World War II. He learned about exciting advances in genetics in the 1950s. He also learned about the new way of testing blood, called hemoglobin electrophoresis. He combined his interests in biochemistry, genetics and geography into a landmark project. His plan when he set out on that university expedition in 1949 was to create a map of African blood groups based on the blood samples he would collect, and through it to stake out the long, slow trajectory of human evolution. As so often happens, however, he got distracted by a different question. Just before Allison went back to Africa, a hematologist alerted him to the puzzle then posed by sickle cell disease. At the time, scientists could not explain why this disease remained in the African population even though it killed its victims before they reached puberty—in other words, before they were able to pass on the faulty gene.

Allison decided to test for sickle trait while he was collecting blood samples from people in different parts of East Africa and Central Africa. Almost immediately, he noticed the odd distribution of the sickle cell gene—it was much more common on the coast and around Lake Victoria than in the highlands. "Half the young children in the pediatric wards in Malindi and-Mombasa on the coast, and in Kisumu near the lake, had sickle cell disease," he said, and it was usually fatal. He was distressed by what he saw, perhaps because it reminded him of his own bouts of sickness when he was infected with malaria as a boy. But that reminder, too, was serendipitous, because now the various elements of the answer were floating in his subconscious. The eureka moment came during a party in the Ngong Hills to mark the end of the expedition—the sickle cell gene, he realized, was most prevalent in the hot, humid areas where the malaria parasite thrived.

Allison knew that to have sickle cell disease, a person must have two copies of the sickle cell gene. Those who have only one copy are merely carriers. It occurred to him that the gene might have remained in the pool because carriers had an evolutionary advantage over non-carriers—they were protected against that other African scourge, malaria.

He had to wait four frustrating years to return to East Africa to test his hunch, but return he did, as a qualified medic who had worked hard at his parasitology in the interim, travelling this time on a "sickle cell safari" across East Africa from the Semliki Forest of western Uganda, down past Lake Victoria and the highlands of Kenya and Tanzania to the coast. A crucial piece of equipment was a battery-operated microscope inside his tent. Allison managed to test 5,000 East Africans, representing three countries and more than thirty different tribes.

STATISTICS ON SICKLE TRAIT LEADS TO AN IDEA

Borrowing the concept of balanced polymorphism from his teacher E.B. Ford at Oxford, Allison, hypothesized that sickle cell trait offered protection against malaria. People with sickle trait did not catch malaria infection as often, but, when they did have malaria, the infection was less severe. This meant that children with sickle trait were less likely to die of malaria, and then they could survive to adulthood to pass along the protective sickle trait gene to some of their children.

So the hypothesis also meant that the sickle gene would be more common in regions with more intense malaria, because children with sickle trait have an advantage in combatting the effects of malaria over individuals with normal hemoglobin (i.e., HbAA).

When the carriers of an abnormal gene have a survival advantage over the rest of the population, the scientific situation is known as balanced polymorphism. Balanced polymorphism works to maintain a high frequency of people with one copy of the recessive mutant gene (in this case, many people with sickle trait), even though having two copies of the mutant gene causes major health problems (in this case, sickle cell disease).

Allison took more blood samples, comparing the parasite loads in carriers and non-carriers of the sickle cell gene, and the fruits of his efforts were published in a now-famous series of three papers in 1954.

> (1) incidence of the [sickle] trait in East Africa has recently been investigated in detail (Allison, 1954), and found to vary in accordance with the above hypothesis. High frequencies are observed among the tribes living in regions where malaria is hyperendemic (for example, around Lake Victoria and in the Eastern Coastal Belt), whereas low frequencies occur consistently in the malaria-free or epidemic zones (for example, the Kigezi district of Uganda; the Kenya Highlands; and the Kilimanjaro, Mount Meru, and Usumbara regions of Tanganyika). This difference is often independent of ethnic and linguistic grouping: thus, the incidence of the sickle cell trait among Bantu-speaking tribes ranges from 0 (among the Kamba, Chagga, etc.) to 40% (among the Amba, Simbiti, etc.).
>
> —Allison A.C. (1954) "Protection afforded by sickle-cell trait against subtertian malarial infection." *British Medical Journal* 4857: 290–294

The theory was greeted with skepticism at first, but by the time he was invited to present it at the prestigious Cold Spring Harbor Laboratory in New

Malaria resistance is provided by sickle trait, an inherited condition that is common in areas with a lot of malaria infection.

Besides sickle hemoglobin, other abnormal hemoglobins are frequently inherited by people in West Africa, Asia, and other places with a lot of malaria: hemoglobin C, hemoglobin E, beta thalassemia, alpha thalassemia, and others. Most of these hemoglobins have now been shown to provide some resistance to malaria.

A chemical called G-6PD is deficient in the red blood cells of many people from these areas also. This inherited deficiency can cause problems of red blood cell breakdown after exposure to an oxidant chemical such as mothballs (napthalene) or sulfa antibiotics. G-6PD deficiency also provides some resistance against malaria infection.

Another red blood cell abnormality called Southeast Asian ovalocytosis also provides some resistance against malaria infection. So it looks like many kinds of red blood cell problems can be linked to malaria resistance. However, when there is no malaria around, the red blood cells are still abnormal and can sometimes cause problems that are treated by a blood specialist (hematologist). Some people say that hematologists would not be in business if it wasn't for malaria, because there would be much fewer abnormal red blood cell conditions.

York later that year, it had the scientific establishment's seal of approval. Allison showed maps to demonstrate how the distribution of malaria and the frequency of sickle trait across Africa match closely. The frequency of the sickle trait was 20% to 40% in East African regions with high rates of malaria infection, but sickle trait was rare or zero in the highlands of Kenya, Uganda, and Tanzania. Other studies have showed that abnormal hemoglobins are common in other groups of people with intense malaria exposure, including pockets of Greece and India. This work helped to revive an idea of Louis Pasteur's, that susceptibility to infectious diseases is inherited.

In the five decades since Allison published his theory, evidence has accumulated to support it. When studies were restricted to young people, the hypothesis held—the sickle cell trait did offer protection to children, but not to adults, since they were unable to develop antibodies to the malarial parasite.

Studies have shown that African Americans, who have lived in malaria-free areas for as long as ten generations, have lower sickle cell gene frequencies than Africans—and the frequencies have dropped more than those of other, less harmful African genes.

Similarly, the sickle cell gene is less common among blacks in Curaçao, a malaria-free island in the Caribbean, than in Suriname, a neighboring country where malaria is rampant, even though the ancestors of both populations came from the same region of Africa.

HOW DOES SICKLE TRAIT PROVIDE PROTECTION AGAINST MALARIA?

At the time, Dr. Tony Allison did not know how the presence of sickle cell hemoglobin gave selective protection against malaria, but the connection seemed clear to him.

Later research showed that sickle trait makes the blood resist malaria infection in several different ways, most of which stem from the abnormal sickle hemoglobin breaking down more easily inside the red blood cell, to create the fragment molecule called hemichrome.

Hemichrome creates an oxidant stress that is hostile to the malaria parasite inside of the red blood cell in many ways:

1. It changes the transport molecules (actin filaments) that the malaria parasite uses to move itself around within the red blood cell.
2. It alters the malaria parasite's exit sites (knob-shaped structures called PfEMP-1).
3. It changes the red blood cell stiffness and surface properties to make the red blood cell less likely to stick to the blood vessel wall in small venules, which is where the malaria parasite prefers to live, and instead be removed from the bloodstream.

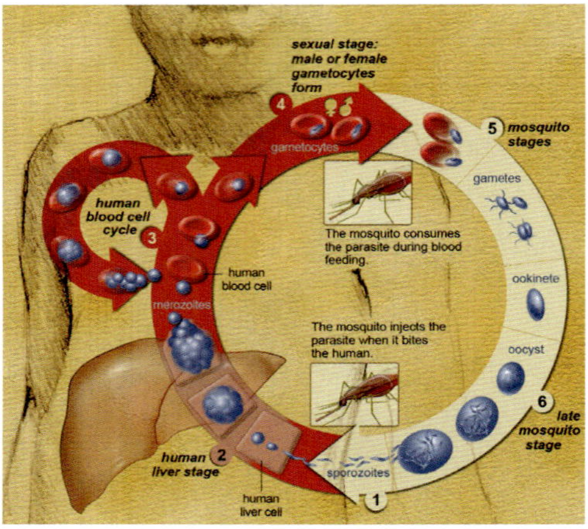

National Institutes of Health

Life cycle of the malaria parasite

WHAT KIND OF DISEASE IS MALARIA?

Malaria is an infection with a parasite with the scientific name *Plasmodium*. The malaria parasite is transmitted by the bite of female mosquitoes. It needs to spend part of its life cycle inside the mosquito and part of its life cycle inside the human red blood cell.

The malaria parasites grow and reproduce inside the red blood cell, burst the red blood cell and then enter other red blood cells. After a few cycles of living in red blood cells in the human, the parasites move into the next phase of their life cycle and change to a different form that can be picked up by another mosquito. The parasite has a favorite family of mosquito: *Anopheles* mosquito. That mosquito brings some of the malaria parasite to the next person, and the parasite's life cycle continues. The person infected with malaria can have high fevers, and periods when the urine is very dark brown whenever a lot of red blood cells are broken by parasites. Swelling of the brain, spleen, and other organs can make the person very sick or even cause them to die.

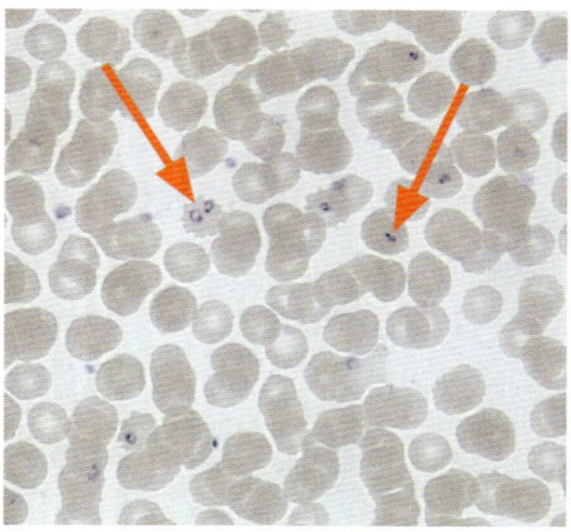

Michael Zahniser

The blue spots are malaria parasites.

The malaria parasites can be seen inside the red blood cells using a microscope to look at a drop of blood on a glass slide. In this microscopic view of human blood (100x magnification, treated with hematoxylin, a special stain), malaria parasites can be seen inside some red blood cells. About six red blood cells each contain one or two parasites stained blue. At this life-stage they are knobby ring-shaped structures, called male and female gametocytes (stage four in the life-cycle figure above).

WHY IS MALARIA COMMON IN SOME PLACES AND NOT SEEN IN OTHER PLACES?

Malaria's life cycle depends on having both humans and mosquitoes close to each other. Warm, wet areas have plenty of mosquitoes. Mosquito breeding sites are found anywhere fresh water collects—a swamp, a rice paddy, a drainage ditch along the road, a muddy footprint in the road, a few spoonfuls of water trapped by the leaves of a plant, a well, a fountain, and even the rainwater pooled in an old rubber tire or empty can. Dry deserts and high mountains have very few mosquitoes. Mosquitoes also do not live well during cold winters.

HOW DOES SICKLE TRAIT PROVIDE PROTECTION AGAINST MALARIA?

The abnormal hemoglobin breaks down more easily inside the red blood cell and creates oxidant stress that is hostile to the malaria parasite inside of the red blood cell. The oxidant stress also changes the transport molecules that the malaria parasite uses to exit the red blood cell and makes the red blood cells stiffer and more likely to be removed early from the bloodstream.

HOW CAN MALARIA BE TREATED OR PREVENTED?

Humans can stop mosquitoes from biting during the night by sleeping under mosquito netting. This netting has tiny holes that are too small for mosquitoes to fit through but big enough to allow the sleeper to have air and light. The bed nets can also be treated with insecticide. The bed net can be used every night for a long time, but you have to be careful not to tear it and make a hole large enough to let a mosquito through.

Humans can stop mosquitoes from growing by covering small puddles or ponds of water, because mosquitoes must use water surfaces as breeding space. People can also stop mosquitoes by spraying insect killers on water that has the young forms of the mosquito (larva).

Malaria can also be treated or prevented with anti-malaria medicine. Travelers going to a malaria zone should use mosquito repellant spray and mosquito netting, and take anti-malaria medicine that is suitable for the specific type of malaria common in that region. Some older anti-malaria medicines are quinine and chloroquine. Newer medicines include mefloquine, primaquine, artemesinin, doxycycline, and halofantrine. Scientists are trying to develop an effective vaccine against malaria.

THE TUSKEGEE AIRMEN AND DR. MARCHBANKS HELP PROVE THAT PEOPLE WITH SICKLE TRAIT CAN BE PILOTS

The Tuskegee Airmen were famous for their service record of being "first" and "best"—first African-American military pilots, best record as escort fighters and first to shoot down a German jet fighter. They overcame a lot of prejudice and adversity to prove that African Americans can be fighter pilots, and they helped break the color barrier in the United States military.

About 450 Tuskegee fighter pilots flew more than 15,000 missions over North Africa and Europe during World War II.

Nicknamed the "Red Tails" because of the distinctive paint on their planes, they shot down more than 110 enemy aircraft and destroyed hundreds

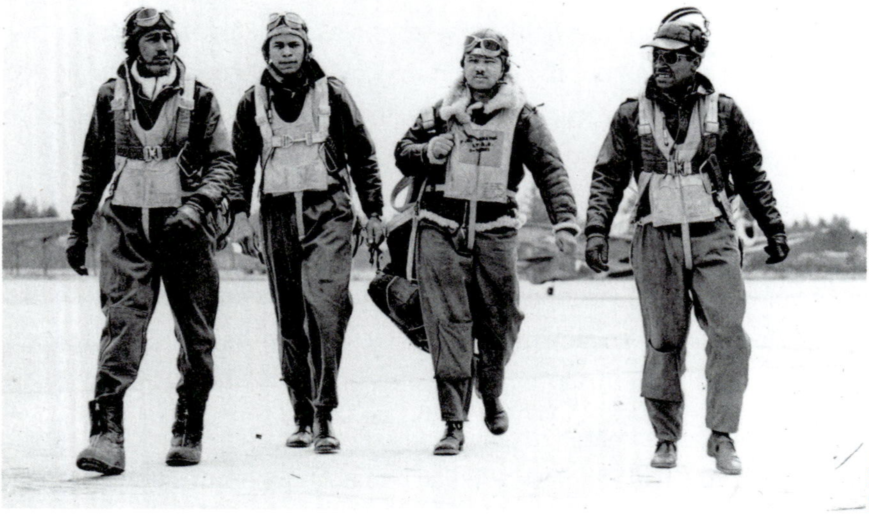

U.S. Air Force

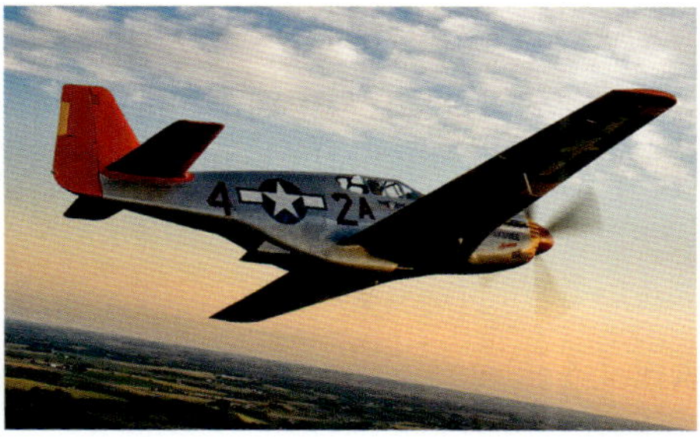

more on the ground, along with dozens of railroad cars, boats and barges. Impressed by their skill, bomber crews asked for them as escorts.

The fliers collectively earned close to 1,000 medals, including Distinguished Flying Crosses, Presidential Unit Citations, Bronze Stars and Purple Hearts. More than sixty pilots were killed in action, and thirty more were shot down and captured. Their commander, Benjamin O. Davis, Jr., later became a four-star general.

Did you know that they also helped to prove that people with sickle trait can be pilots? In 1942 Dr. Vance H. Marchbanks, Jr. had completed the Army Air Corps course in aviation medicine and was rated an aviation medical examiner. He was assigned to the station hospital at the Tuskegee Army Airfield then transferred as a major with the 332nd Fighter Group, known as the Tuskegee Airmen, to Selfridge Field, Michigan. They went on to serve in North Africa and Italy, and some of their stories are shown in the recent movie *Red Tails*. Marchbanks was the group's flight surgeon during World War II campaigns in Italy, becoming one of the first Black American flight surgeons and the first in the Air Force's medical service. He earned a Bronze Star.

In 1973, a committee of scientists recommended that people with sickle trait could serve in the military except for flight duty as pilots and co-pilots. In 1979, the Air Force Academy in Colorado Springs, Colorado, expelled Stephen Pullens and five other Black cadets after a week of courses at the Academy on the grounds that the high altitude of the Academy (7,000 feet) would be harmful to their health because they have sickle trait. They filed a class-action suit against the Air Force. But there was very little evidence that pilots with sickle trait really could function at the low oxygen at high altitude. Since people with sickle trait were being barred from training as pilots, how would anybody get this proof? Dr. Marchbanks thought of a way.

Although he had retired from military service along with his comrades in the 332nd Fighter Group, Marchbanks would ask the retired Tuskegee Airmen to volunteer for one more duty. He guessed that some of the Tuskegee Airmen who had already served very successfully as combat pilots would turn out to have sickle trait.

A blood sample on each man could be tested to see who had sickle trait, and then their service records would be examined for any sign of weakness or problems at high altitude. Would their flying records prove that people with sickle trait could be great pilots, or would the ones with sickle trait actually have records showing difficulty with high altitude performance? Would these retired pilots be willing to put their service records to the test? Or would they say, "It's not my job anymore, I'm retired now, I have no more need to prove myself, I'll just mind my own business and not try to challenge the military's policy of discharging men who carry the sickle-cell anemia trait"?

One hundred fifty-four Tuskegee Airmen volunteered for Marchbanks' study, and he tested their blood for sickle trait. He compared the flying records of those with and without sickle trait and showed that the ten pilots with sickle trait had no problems in combat performance. One pilot with sickle trait had 600 hours of combat experience with no problems. The only pilot who had any episode of losing consciousness at high altitude was a person without sickle trait. This landmark study, published in the article "Sickle Cell Trait and the Black Airman," helped prove that not everyone who carries the trait has the disease, and that sickle trait did not prevent these ten Tuskegee Airmen from serving as combat military pilots. Marchbanks convinced military authorities not to end the careers of Black cadets in the Air Force who had the sickle-cell trait. The Air Force changed the policy about sickle trait pilots in May 1981, just one year after Marchbanks published his study on the Tuskegee Airmen.

Many people have sickle cell trait or disease, just like you and some of the Tuskegee Airmen. But with healthy practices, medical attention, and continuing advances in science, you can live a full, active life and achieve the dreams you set for yourself.

RESOURCES

WEB SITES FOR EVERYONE

https://www.cdc.gov/ncbddd/sicklecell/l

https://www.nhlbi.nih.gov/health/sickle-cell-disease

https://sicklecellcenters.org/member_centers

WEB SITES FOR PARENTS

https://cscfkids.org/

SMARTPHONE APPS

Pinpoint™—Using gaming technology and developed by expert clinicians and parents of teens with sickle cell disease, Pinpoint™ is an evidence-based mobile health app that provides a safe, convenient tool for teens to learn about, track, assess, and communicate about their sickle cell pain with medical providers and parents. Pinpoint™ works on any smartphone or smart mobile device and pain assessment reports can be shared electronically with parents and/or providers through the app with the teen's consent. Visit *www.hpcinternationalinc.com/products/pinpoint* for more information and to download the app. *Available in 2023 for Apple and Android devices.*

Voice Crisis Alert V2 allows you to track your symptoms and pain and share them with your family members and healthcare providers. *Available in the App Store and Google Play Store.*

Sickle-O-Scope is a diary to record your symptoms, with visualizations of your condition. You can share the data you collect with your healthcare provider. *Available in the App Store and Google Play Store.*

SickleBuddy is an app for children to learn and live with sickle cell disease. *Available in the App Store.*

SCD Toolbox is an app for adults and includes medical guides. *Available in the App Store.*

SCD Share is an app to increase awareness and knowledge of sickle disease. *Available in the App Store.*

NON-FICTION BOOKS WRITTEN FOR YOUNG PEOPLE

Hope and Destiny Jr. Workbook by Lewis Hsu, MD. A streamlined version of *Hope and Destiny Jr.*, plus some added educational puzzles, written for children in their "tweens." *https://hpcinternationalinc.com/Bookstore*

My Sickle Cell Journal by Hilton Publishing helps sickle cell patients to write about their thoughts and feelings. It has also been designed to serve as a useful tool for doctors by prompting patients to record medication side effects, their personal experience with the disease, and even questions they want to ask at their next office visit. *https://hpcinternationalinc.com/Bookstore*

Sickle Cell Anemia (What Does It Mean to Have?) by Heinemann (2005)

Sickle Cell Disease by Susan Dudley Gold and Lillian McMahon (2001)

Sickle Cell Anemia by Alvin Silverstein, Virginia B. Silverstein, & Laura Silverstein Nunn (1997)

FICTION BOOKS WRITTEN FOR YOUNG PEOPLE

Sickle Cell Superheroes by Destiny Van Sciver is a sweet fictional story about a young girl showing bravery, strength and determination to live her life to the fullest despite the obstacles she sometimes faces with her blood disorder. This book is a perfect resource for patients and families in hematology departments and sickle cell clinics, and makes a wonderful addition to any school library, to teach elementary-aged students what it's like living with SCD. *https://hpcinternationalinc.com/Bookstore*

Now You See Me, Now You Don't by Jan Reed-Givhan

Locomotion (Coretta Scott King Author Honor Books) by Jacqueline Woodson (2003)

Puzzles by Dava Walker (1996)

Big Man and the Burnout by Clayton Bess (1985)

NON-FICTION BOOKS WRITTEN FOR PARENTS

Hope and Destiny: A Patient's and Parent's Guide to Sickle Cell Disease and Sickle Cell Trait—6th Edition by Allan Platt, PA-C, Lewis Hsu, M.D., and James Eckman, MD provides clear-cut and in-depth information for the more than 100,000 Americans living with sickle cell disease. *https://hpcinternationalinc.com/Bookstore*

Sickle What? by Lisa Rose breaks down complex medical concepts and terminology into simple, easy to understand language. Focusing on new parents facing a diagnosis of SCD, *Sickle What?* arms families with the knowledge they need to understand and manage this painful disease. *https://hpcinternationalinc.com/Bookstore*

Living Well With Sickle Cell: A Handbook for Parents is written in a friendly, understandable method specifically for new parents and contains practical information and resources for daily life with SCD. By Andrea Matthews and the Children's Sickle Cell Foundation. *https://hpcinternationalinc.com/Bookstore*

Sickle Cell Disease: A Booklet for Patients, Parents and the Community by Dr. Adlette Inati Khoriaty, available at *https://thalassaemia.org.cy/publications/tif-publications/sickle-cell-disease-2008/*

Sickle by Dominique Friend

I Only Cry At Night by P. Allen Jones

The Stranger Within Me by Shirley Renee

MOVIES THAT HAVE CHARACTERS WITH SICKLE CELL DISEASE

Spilled Milk (2018), directed by Jaqai Mickelsen

Documentary to raise awareness about sickle cell disease through the lens of a close friendship between Omar and Jaqai, and taking steps towards eliminating stigma of sickle cell. Omar is somebody that Jaqai has always held in high esteem. He is intelligent, even-tempered, funny, and has great penmanship. The title of the film is a reminder of what Omar and Jaqai arrived at together, that you can cry over spilled milk or embrace what you have.

Walk by Faith (2014), starring Dominyck McCargo, Trina Brown, Bradley Smith, Rochelle Ojeda
Rating: TV-PG

Genre: Drama

A teenager lives with the painful effects of sickle cell anemia then begins the process of seeking a donor for a bone marrow transplant.

A Warm December (1973), starring Esther Anderson and Sidney Poitier
Rating: PG

Genre: Drama, Medical Drama

The second directorial effort from Academy Award-winning actor Sidney Poitier, this romantic drama is about widowed American doctor Matt Younger (Poitier) who travels to London with his daughter, Stefanie (Yvette Curtis). There, he meets Catherine (Esther Anderson), the daughter of African Ambassador George Oswandu (Earl Cameron). A romance develops between them, and Dr. Younger realizes that the strange men that follow Catherine around have been hired by her father in order to keep an eye on her sickle cell anemia. –Andrea LeVasseur

Nurse.Fighter.Boy (2009), starring Clark Johnson, Daniel J. Gordon, David Collins, Karen LeBlanc, Walter Borden
Genre: Drama

Nurse.Fighter.Boy is an urban love story about the soul of a mother, the heart of a fighter, and the faith of a child. Jude is a single mother who descends from a long line of Jamaican caregivers. Silence is a "past his prime" boxer who fights illegally to survive. Ciel is a boy who delves into music, conjuring dreams for his mother. During the last week of summer, a late-night brawl finds the fighter in the nurse's care causing their three fates to be forever entwined.

GLOSSARY

504 plan—a plan created for a student with a disability, allowing that student to continue learning among his or her classmates with certain changes to the learning environment, such as extra bathroom breaks or allowing the student to keep water at his or her desk.

Acute chest syndrome—When sickled red blood cells block blood flow to the lungs. This can cause chest pain, shortness of breath, and cough. It is treated in the hospital with blood transfusions. It can be prevented with incentive spirometry (a "blow bottle").

Acute hemolytic reaction—a medical emergency occurring within 24 hours of receiving a blood transfusion, during which the recipient's body attacks and destroys the newly transfused donor blood cells. See also delayed hemolytic reaction.

Adakveo®—Crizanlizumab-tmca was approved in 2019 to reduce the frequency of pain crisis in sickle cell patients 16 and older. It is marketed in the United States as Adakveo®. Crizanlizumab is a humanized monoclonal antibody that binds to P-selectin and reduces binding to the lining of blood vessels platelets, red cells, and white blood cells. Binding of these cells to blood vessels lining and each other is thought to start pain crises by slowing blood flow and blocking blood vessels.

Advocacy—Health advocacy supports and promotes patient's health care rights. Advocacy activities can also include working to enhance community health, and working to change government policies on making health care available, safe, and with high quality.

Amniocentesis—A test done by taking a small amount of fluid from the womb of a pregnant woman to determine if the baby has sickle cell disease or another genetic problem. This is usually performed when the pregnancy is 15–18 weeks along.

Anemia—A low red blood cell count. Anemia can be caused by many different events, including sickle cell disease.

Antigens—molecules on the surface of a red blood cell that help the body to recognize a foreign cell in the bloodstream. When an antigen finds a cell that should not be there, it signals the body to begin an immune response by creating antibodies to fight off that foreign cell.

Aplastic anemia or aplastic crisis—Decreased red blood cell count due to the bone marrow factory temporarily shutting down. The most common cause is a virus called Parvovirus B19.

Autologous blood transfusions—transfusions using blood you have donated yourself

Automated erythrocytapheresis—also known as automated red blood cell exchange. In this procedure, blood is drawn with a needle or catheter, then put into an apheresis machine. This machine separates the red blood cells from the other parts of the blood (white cells, platelets, and plasma). The separated red cells are discarded, and the remaining parts of the blood are mixed with healthy red cells from a donor and then returned to the patient. This procedure can help patients avoid iron overload from blood transfusions.

Avascular necrosis (AVN)—Bones, like other organs in the body, need blood to stay alive and healthy. Unfortunately, sickle red blood cells can sometimes block the blood supply to the round part of either the hip or shoulder bone. This lack of blood flow causes the bone to die, resulting in long-term hip or shoulder pain. The normal joint is a ball-and-socket. The damaged joint might have a flattened ball that does not fit well into the socket anymore, which is called avascular necrosis (AVN)

Bilirubin—A yellow-orange chemical produced from the breakdown of hemoglobin, when red blood cells break down.

Blood phenotype—the pattern of all antigens or surface molecules on a red blood cell.

Bone marrow—Inside of your big bones, the marrow has cells that can make red blood cells, white blood cells, and platelets. Bone marrow is soft and spongy , and some people call the marrow the "blood factory."

Bone marrow transplant—A procedure that kills the existing bone marrow production and plants donor (usually a matched brother or sister) marrow by transfusion. The bone marrow begins to make blood cells according to the genetic code of the donor. This has cured over 600 sickle cell patients.

Carrier—One who inherits only one gene for a genetic problem like sickle cell. Usually there are no symptoms, and the carrier will never have the disease. Two carriers of sickle trait have a 25% risk of having a child with sickle cell disease.

Chemotherapy—a type of medication usually used to treat cancer. In sickle cell disease, chemotherapy can be used to wipe out your bone marrow before you receive a stem cell or bone marrow transplant.

Chorionic villus sampling (CVS)—This is a procedure to determine if a baby in the womb has a genetic disease like sickle cell. It is done when the pregnancy is 10–12 weeks along. A catheter or needle is used to get a sample of the placenta for testing.

Chromosome—The DNA code for all the parts of the human body. Each person has 46 individual chromosomes in cells, 23 donated from each parent. Chromosome 11 is where the sickle cell mutation occurs.

Complete blood count (CBC)—A blood test that gives information about how many red cells, white cells, and platelets a person has in their bloodstream.

Cord blood—This is the blood remaining in the umbilical cord and placenta after a baby is born and the cord is cut. This blood is rich in stem cells that can be saved and used in transplants.

Delayed hemolytic reaction—This type of reaction happens when the body slowly attacks antigens (other than ABO antigens) on the transfused blood cells. The blood cells are broken down days or weeks after the transfusion. There are usually no symptoms, but the transfused red blood cells are destroyed and the patient's red blood cell count falls. In rare cases, the kidneys may be affected and treatment may be needed. One way this might show up is through brown urine that is the color of cola. People do not usually have this type of reaction unless they have had transfusions in the past. If you do have this type of reaction, you'll need special blood testing before any more blood can be transfused. Units of blood that do not have the antigen that the body is attacking must be used.

Endari® (L-glutamine)—L-glutamine oral powder is a new medication for sickle cell disease. It was approved by the FDA in 2017 and first entered the US market in 2018 under the brand name Endari®. It works primarily by boosting the antioxidant properties of the red blood cell, helping the body fight oxidant damage and cut down on inflammation.

Enuresis—the medical term for wetting the bed, a common side effect of having sickle cell disease due to effects of the disorder on the kidneys

Erythrocytapheresis—see automated erythrocytapheresis

FARMS—An acronym to help you remember ways you can manage your sickle cell symptoms: **F**luids/Fever (drink plenty of liquids and manage fevers), **A**ir (get enough oxygen and be careful at high altitudes), **R**est (get plenty of sleep), **M**edication (e.g. penicillin, hydroxyurea, folic acid), and **S**ituations to avoid (e.g. stress, extreme temperatures, dehydration, drugs and alcohol).

Folic acid or folate—A B vitamin necessary for making new red blood cells. It also acts as a vasodilator, which allows your blood to flow more freely through small blood vessels, and it helps homocysteine level, which may reduce your risk of complications, such as stroke, leg ulcers, and heart attack. Most sickle cell patients should take 1 mg a day. It is found in green, leafy vegetables, fruits, and whole grains.

Gallbladder—A pouch in the right upper abdomen under the liver. It stores bile to help digest fats in the diet. The gallbladder can be removed if it is full of gallstones and causing problems.

Gallstones—Too much bilirubin from red blood cell breakdown can cause stones to form in the gallbladder. This can cause pain in the right upper abdomen, nausea, and indigestion when eating fatty foods.

Genes—These are the basic units of inheritance. They are located on chromosomes.

Gene therapy—Treatment that will change the genetic defect or the gene product (hemoglobin) in sickle cell disease. The first experimental studies of gene therapy for human sickle cell disease started in 2014.

Glutamine—Glutamine is an amino acid, and it has recently been approved as a treatment for sickle cell disease. It's currently available under the brand name Endari. Glutamine works primarily by boosting the antioxidant properties of the red blood cell. Antioxidants help the body minimize oxidant damage.

GVHD (Graft-versus-host disease)—GVHD can occur after a bone marrow or stem cell transplant when someone receives bone marrow tissue or cells from a donor and the donor's immune cells attack some of your organs. Before a transplant, tissue and cells from possible donors are checked to see how closely they match the person having the transplant. The closer the match, the less likely GVHD is to occur. Treatments to help prevent GVHD may include immunosuppressants, antibiotics and sometimes steroids. Symptoms of GVHD normally occur within 12 months of the transplant and can include skin rash, nausea, diarrhea, jaundice, dry eyes, dry mouth, weight loss and many others.

Hand-foot syndrome or dactylitis—Swelling and pain in the hands and feet, usually seen in six-month- to three-year-old sickle cell patients.

Hemoglobin—The protein substance inside the red blood cells that holds and releases oxygen. This is where the sickle mutation occurs.

Hemoglobin AS—This is sickle cell trait. The inheritance of one normal hemoglobin gene and one sickle hemoglobin gene.

Hemoglobin electrophoresis—The blood test that identifies the type of hemoglobins present in the red blood cells.

Hemoglobin S beta thalassemia—This is a type of sickle cell disease in which one inherits an S gene and a beta thalassemia gene from his or her parents. S beta0 thalassemia is more severe than S beta+ thalassemia.

Hemoglobin SC—A type of sickle cell disease in which one inherits an S gene and a C gene from the parents. This causes sickle cell complications, with increased eye and bone problems. Life expectancy is longer than with hemoglobin SS.

Hemoglobin SS—This is called sickle cell anemia and is the most common form of sickle cell disease.

Hemolysis—The breaking apart of red blood cells. Normal red cells last 120 days; sickled red blood cells last about fourteen days.

Hemolytic transfusion reaction—a serious complication that can occur after a blood transfusion. If a patient's blood phenotype is not closely matched to a donor's phenotype, the patient's immune system can attack and destroy the donor cells.

Human leukocyte antigen (HLA) typing —a process used to match patients and donors for blood stem cell transplants. HLA are proteins, or markers, found on most cells in your body. Your immune system uses these markers to recognize which cells belong in your body and which do not. If you need a transplant, your doctor will take a blood sample to test for your HLA type. A close match between your HLA markers and your donor's can reduce the risk that your immune cells will attack your donor's cells (graft rejection) or that your donor's immune cells will attack your body after the transplant (graft versus host disease, or GVHD).

Hydroxyurea—The first medication for sickle cell disease that increases fetal hemoglobin. It reduces pain events by one half, the need for hospital admissions, absences from school or work, the need for blood transfusions—

and it prolongs the lifespan.

Hyphema—If an eye injury causes bleeding in the eye, sickle trait blood cells can become trapped in the eye in a condition called hyphema. This blood can quickly cause vision loss if it is not flushed out. An eye specialist should be notified immediately about sickle trait and serious eye injury. The treatment can include close monitoring of the bleeding eye and eye pressure for several days.

Individualized education program (IEP)—a plan created for a student with a disability, giving that student help through special education services, which are provided by the student's school district.

Intravenous (IV) line—A small plastic catheter placed in a vein to allow water, blood, or medication to enter the blood stream directly.

Jaundice—A yellow color in the white part (sclera) of the eye produced by increased bilirubin in the blood. Usually caused by increased red blood cell breakdown in sickle cell patients. Jaundice is not harmful and shouldn't be concerning.

Leukoreduction—the process of filtering out white blood cells from donated blood. Leukoreduced blood can reduce risks to the blood recipient, including fever after transfusion, poor response to platelet transfusion, and the spread of certain viruses from the donor to the recipient.

LOCATES—An acronym to help you remember how to record your pain: **L**ocation (where does it hurt?), **O**ther symptoms, **C**haracter (is the pain deep, burning?), **A**ggravating and alleviating things (what makes the pain worse or better?), **T**iming (when did it start?), **E**nvironment and effect (what was happening when the pain started, and how does it affect you?), and **S**everity.

Magnetic resonance imaging (MRI)—Taking pictures of the brain or other organs of the body with a large magnet-based device.

Malaria—an infection with a parasite with the scientific name *Plasmodium*. The malaria parasite is transmitted by the bite of female mosquitoes. It needs to spend part of its life cycle inside the mosquito and part of its life cycle inside the human red blood cell. The malaria parasites grow and reproduce inside the red blood cell, burst the red blood cell and then enter other red blood cells. After a few cycles of living in red blood cells in the human, the parasites move into the next phase of their life cycle and change to a different form that can be picked up by another mosquito. The parasite has a favorite family of mosquito: *Anopheles* mosquito. That mosquito brings some of the malaria parasite to the next person, and the parasite's life cycle continues. The person infected with malaria can have high fevers, and periods when the urine is very dark brown whenever a lot of red blood cells are broken by parasites. Swelling of the brain, spleen, and other organs can make the person very sick or even cause them to die.

Non-ablative bone marrow transplant—The newest transplant method for sickle cell is the non-ablative approach. It is also called *partial mixed chimerism*. With this method, enough donor marrow is transplanted to the patient to produce normal red blood cells. The better red blood cells produced by the donor marrow have a longer lifespan than sickle red blood cells, which will allow the healthy cells to eventually become the majority of the circulating red blood cells.

Osteomyelitis—Bone infection

Oxbryta®—Voxelotor was approved by the FDA in 2019 and it is marketed in the United States as Oxbryta®. It works by binding to the sickle hemoglobin and increasing the tightness of the bond of oxygen (the oxygen affinity). This reduces sickling and the breakdown of red cells (hemolysis). The main clinical benefit is an increase in hemoglobin level and reduced markers of hemolysis. It may also improve blood flow by making red cells more flexible.

Oxidant damage—Oxidant damage is the same thing that causes iron to rust and sliced apples and avocados to turn brown, and in the human body it increases the risk of cancer, heart disease, and stroke. Sickled red cells have more oxidant damage than other red cells. By boosting the antioxidant properties in red blood cells, glutamine helps the body fight oxidant damage and cut down on inflammation.

Pain episode or "crisis"—Pain in the bones and muscles where blood flow has been blocked by sickled red blood cells.

Paxlovid™—Nirmatrelvir/ritonavir, sold under the brand name Paxlovid, is a co-packaged oral medication, developed by Pfizer and used as a treatment for COVID-19. It contains the antiviral medications nirmatrelvir and ritonavir.

Port-a-cath (also other brands like InfusaPort)—An under-the-skin port that requires only a one-time needle stick that allows long-term painless access to sample venous blood, and/or to give IV fluids and medications.

Prenatal testing—ways to check a pregnant woman to determine if the baby has sickle cell disease or another genetic problem. Here are 2 common ways: Chorionic villus sampling (CVS) is done when the pregnancy is 10–12 weeks along. A catheter or needle is used to get a sample of the placenta for testing. Amniocentesis is done when the pregnancy is 15–18 weeks along. A sample of fluid is drawn from the womb.

Priapism—A prolonged painful erection of the penis from trapped sickled red blood cells.

Pulmonary hypertension—The condition in which the lungs' blood vessels are abnormally tight and raise the blood pressure there.

Reticulocyte count or retics—The count of brand new red blood cells just released from the bone marrow factory. It is the best indicator of how the bone marrow factory is producing red cells.

Retina—The back of the eye, where light is detected. The blood vessels of the retina can be weakened or blocked by sickle red blood cells. A retina exam with (eyedrops to dilate the pupils) should be done every year for teens and adults. This can lead to bleeding in the eyeball, and loss of vision.

Retinopathy—damage to the back of the eye, which controls your vision. People can develop different types of retinopathy for various reasons. Sickle cell disease can cause a specific type of retinopathy called sickle cell retinopathy. In the early stages of retinopathy, your vision might be perfect.

However, retinopathy often gets worse, causing vision problems and even blindness. Fortunately, retinopathy can usually be treated by laser surgery before it causes vision problems.

Sepsis—a condition in which bacteria in the blood triggers an inflammation response throughout the body. Sepsis can be life-threatening and requires immediate medical attention.

Spleen—An organ in the left upper area of the stomach that helps filter germs from the blood stream.

Splenic sequestration—Blocked blood flow from sickled red blood cells in the spleen or liver. Blood can flow in, but it cannot flow out. This causes weakness, abdominal pain, and swelling of the liver or spleen.

Sickle cell nephropathy—Sickle red blood cells can damage the kidney so that it is unable to filter your blood properly. This kidney damage is called sickle cell nephropathy. The first sign of this damage is protein in the urine (proteinuria). People with early sickle cell nephropathy have no symptoms, but they can later develop renal failure, which means that the kidneys no longer work. Renal failure can cause dangerous levels of different electrolytes in the blood since the blood is not properly filtered. People with renal failure must go on dialysis or have a kidney transplant.

Stroke—Blocked blood flow to an area of the brain that can cause weakness, numbness, trouble speaking, or trouble thinking. Stroke is a medical emergency.

Transcranial Doppler (TCD)—a special ultrasound device that uses painless sound waves to check for blocked blood flow in the brain. "Transcranial" means that the ultrasound waves go through the skull to capture the speed of blood flow. This test can identify children at greatest risk of having a stroke. It is also known as sickle stroke screen.

Vaso-occlusive pain—unpredictable severe pain, which is a classic symptom of sickle cell disease. It can be triggered by dehydration, exhaustion, infection, low oxygen, emotional stress, change of weather, or chilled skin.

Notes

Sometimes I wish I could play sports, but being involved in Student Council allows me to help others and that's quite fulfilling. ***—Ania, Teen***

I cope by eating healthy and knowing my physical and mental limits—because stress can affect me too."

—Sharon, Teen

Tell the world about your experience with SCD. Your story is unique.

—Lisa, parent

I've taught my daughter not to feel sorry for herself because of her disease; everyone deals with some sort of challenge.

—Myesha, parent

Listen to your parents & ask lots of questions.

—Samone, Teen

I keep a journal of notes for each time my son has a crisis to see patterns of when pain appears. This helps us plan better prevention techniques to avoid recurrence of pain.

—Tanya, parent

Sickle cell will not be a stumbling block, but rather consider it a stepping stone to your success story." *—Wola, parent*

Sickle Cell Resources from Hilton Publishing

Since first published, more than 75,000 books from the trusted *HOPE & DESTINY* series have been used by patients, caregivers, family, students, and professionals. Newly revised, the 2023 editions provide the most comprehensive education about SCD available today. Order now at Amazon or www.hpcinternationalinc.com/bookstore

ADULTS

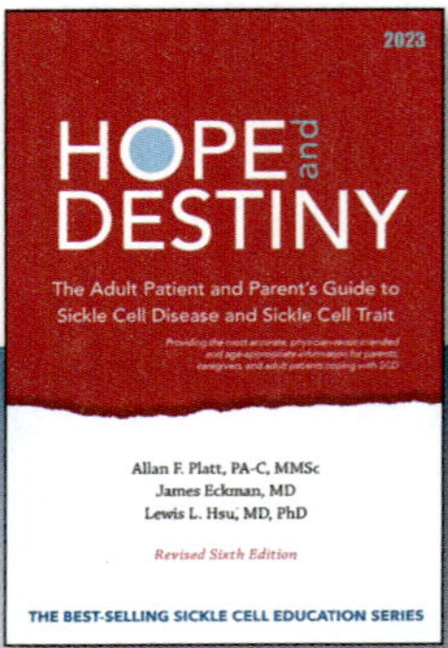

Hope and Destiny: The Adult Patient & Parent's Guide to Sickle Cell Disease

$29.95

978-0-9773160-4-5

TEENS

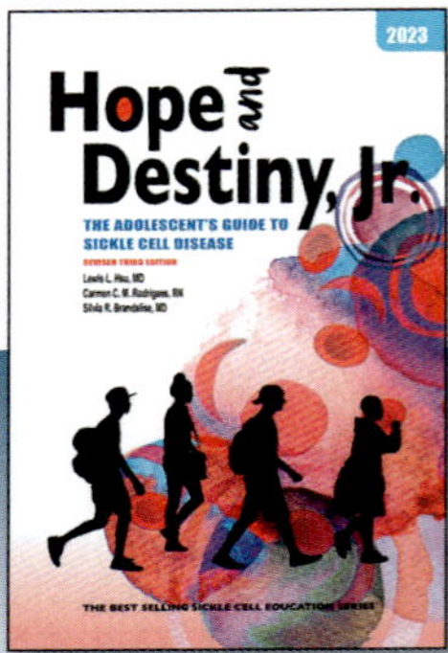

Hope and Destiny Jr.: The Adolescent's Guide to Sickle Cell Disease

$19.95

978-0-9773160-5-2

TEENS

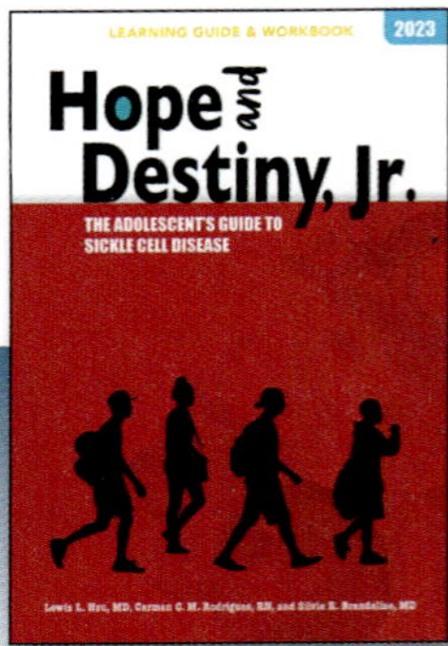

Hope and Destiny Jr.: Adolescent's Learning Guide and Workbook

$13.50

978-0-9773160-6-9

NEW PARENTS

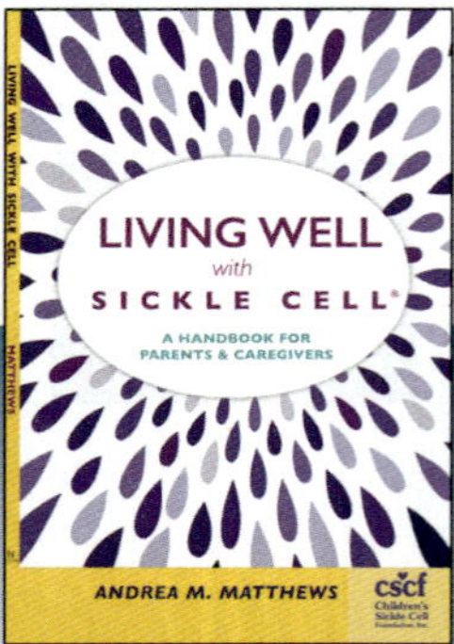

Living Well with Sickle Cell

$18.95

978-0-9983282-4-9

NEW PARENTS

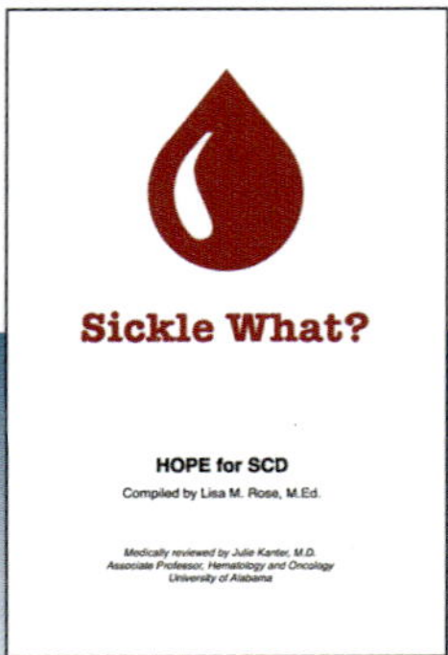

Sickle What?

$17.95

978-0-9773160-1-4

CHILDREN

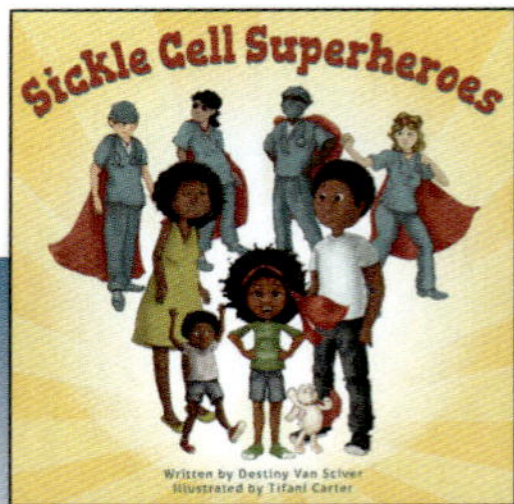

Sickle Cell Superheroes

$15.95

978-0-9773160-2-1